ENDORPHINS

ENDORPHINS

New Waves in Brain Chemistry

JOEL DAVIS

THE DIAL PRESS

Doubleday & Company, Inc.

GARDEN CITY, NEW YORK

1984

Library of Congress Cataloging in Publication Data
Davis, Joel, 1948–
    Endorphins: new waves in brain chemistry.
    1. Endorphins. 2. Brain chemistry. I. Title.
QP552.E53D38 1984   612′.822   83-24017
ISBN 0-385-27856-X

This is for my parents,
Jerry and Toni Davis,
who gave me life;
for Marie, who gives me love;
and for the One who shows me the way.

Contents

Acknowledgments

This book could not have been written without the help and encouragement of a lot of people. First and foremost I must acknowledge the invaluable assistance of Dr. Avram Goldstein, Director of the Addiction Research Foundation, Stanford University, California, and discoverer of beta-endorphin and dynorphin. He ignited my curiosity about these brain chemicals and graciously spent time both on the phone and in person giving me a crash course in neuropharmacology. He answered my questions, drew pictures on blackboards, suggested other people to talk to and gave me much-needed encouragement.

Just as helpful have been several other scientists in the field of brain biochemistry. Roger Guillemin of the Salk Institute for Biological Studies, San Diego, California, was gracious with his time and his answers to questions about his work and its implications. So, too, were Floyd Bloom and George Siggins, now at the Research Institute of Scripps Clinic in La Jolla. Choh Hao Li, Director of the Hormone Research Laboratory, University of California at San Francisco, explained the background and history of his discovery of beta-lipotropin and his subsequent work with different analogues and homologues of opioid peptides. Allan Basbaum and Ellen Glazer at UCSF took time to tell me about pain and endorphins. Roger Nicoll told me about GABA and inhibitory systems in the brain. Ed Herbert, Michael Comb and their associates at the University of Oregon were friendly and patient with me, and tried their best to explain the mysteries of DNA and peptide precursors.

The support and enthusiasm of Ellen Alperstein at East/West

Network for an early article on endorphins encouraged me to poke around some more. As my interest in endorphins grew, Dick Teresi, the executive editor at *Omni,* urged me to make 1982 "the year you write a book." He gave me the name of his literary agent, Barbara Lowenstein, who took a one-page outline, helped me turn it into a thirty-five-page proposal and then sold it in what must be record time. My editor at Dial Press, Jim Fitzgerald, gave me much encouragement throughout the writing of the book. So I owe these four people an enormous debt of gratitude.

Then there was the help and encouragement of a different kind I have gotten from Fathers Mike Baker, Kerry Beaulieu, Jack Christensen, Tim Dyer, and the rest of the infamous Class of '74; from Paul Ford, who warned me about busting deadlines; from the people of St. Mike's in Olympia, especially Sister Mary Giles and Father Jim Jorgenson; from my parents, brothers and sister; from John, Nancy, and Jordy Guth, Jim Docherty, and Joanne, Jennie and Tom McNamara, who gave me a place to stay on my seemingly interminable trips up and down the West Coast; and from the members of the Olympia Chapter of the Northwest Science Fiction Society, for whom nothing seems strange.

Most special thanks go to my wife Marie, who put up with more than a year of obsession, despair, long absences from home, and long nights in front of a word processor. Her reading of preliminary drafts, her patient photocopying of research articles and her constant encouragement made this book possible.

To those who've helped and whose names I have forgotten to mention, my apologies—and my thanks.

And all thanks to θεοΣ ΛοΓοΣ, from whom all words come.

Introduction

The final frontier of knowledge does not lie on the surface of some distant planet, or deep in the fusing interior of the sun. It will not be found at the ever-receding edge of the observable universe, or beneath the sometimes tranquil, sometimes storm-tossed sea surface. The last frontier is not at the center of the earth or even in the intricate workings of the creatures lying at the edge of life and non-life.

The last frontier is within us; it is the fourteen hundred grams of convoluted nerve tissue that lie behind our eyes and between our ears. It is that part of us that enables us to think about it thinking about it.

The human brain is the last frontier.

We tend to think of ourselves as "up there" in the brain, but not all cultures have thought of the brain as the seat of the intellect and the dwelling place of the soul. Some ancients accorded that honor to the liver, others to the heart. Today, though, we think of our body as our body, but of our brain as *us*.

How can we understand or even adequately describe the workings of this intricate mass of living flesh, of blood and fluid, of chemicals and electrical impulses? It is an astounding work of Nature, the brain. Packed into an area smaller than a football are more than a hundred billion nerve cells. There are more brain cells at a dinner for ten than there are stars in the Milky Way galaxy—or galaxies in the observable universe. When we describe the brain and its interconnections as a super telephone switchboard, or a city, or a computer, we do it no justice. No computer has ever come close to the complexity of the brain. It is likely none ever will, despite the claims of AI (artificial intelligence) buffs. For if each nerve cell in the human brain has only two possible states, on or off, then the brain's total capacity is equal to the number two multiplied by itself a hundred *trillion* times.

Almost none of the nerve cells in the brain quite touch each other. Yet connections exist; they are electrochemical connections, and the brain is some kind of electrochemical "computer." Electrical impulses move from nerve cell to nerve cell, carried across the gaps between them by special chemicals.

Sixty years ago no one knew that, no one really knew for sure how the brain worked. Then a series of breakthroughs began which revealed the workings of chemicals in the brain and the body—chemicals which act as messengers carrying information to different parts of the brain and body. A little over ten years ago another brain breakthrough began. It, too, has to do with chemicals in the brain and body. This book is about that new wave of discoveries breaking on the shores of knowledge. It is about the discovery of chemicals in the body called *endorphins.*

Endorphins come in at least three different types and each type has one or more subtypes. There are enkephalins and endorphins and dynorphins. All of them have some amount of opiate activity—they have properties very much like drugs such as heroin or morphine. However, these drugs are "natural." The body makes them for its own use, both in the brain and in the endocrine system of hormones. But they're powerful stuff, these endorphins. At least one kind has shown itself in some tests to be more than seven hundred times as powerful as morphine. For that reason many scientists and researchers think the endorphins are somehow involved in the way we feel pain; in various types of mental illness; and of course in the mechanism of drug addiction and abuse. In the nine years since the first endorphins were discovered some of those possible connections have proved true; others have still to be confirmed; but other endorphin connections have also been uncovered.

Soon after endorphins were discovered they were found to be addictive, as are their more well-known opiate drug cousins. The connection between drug addiction and the endorphins is less straightforward than that of pain, but it is there, and researchers are mapping it out. The results of this work could be a pain-relieving opiate-type drug that is not addictive. But just the opposite possibility also exists: the creation of new and much more powerfully addictive drugs than heroin or methadone.

Dozens of experiments in the last few years confirm the role of endorphins in pain and its regulation. Endorphins are "inhibitory neurotransmitters"—that is, in the brain and nervous system they act to slow down the transmission of information. When each individual in a group of terminal cancer patients received just one injection of a tiny amount of an endorphin, they experienced a profound and long-lasting relief from their pain. When women in labor got injections of endorphins into their lower spinal column, they too got total relief from the pain of labor— and all had normal deliveries of perfectly healthy babies. Other experiments have proved a connection between the action of endorphins and the pain relief of acupuncture.

Some researchers have been looking at possible connections between the endorphins and mental illness, especially schizophrenia. Early experiments suggested endorphins could cure this terrible illness. More recent evidence suggests some schizophrenias may actually be caused by too much endorphin in the brain. Electroconvulsive shock therapy (ECT), though controversial, does often have beneficial effects. And it is often accompanied by changes in the levels of endorphins in people's brain and spinal fluid. Other experiments suggest that the beneficial lithium treatment for manic-depression may somehow be connected to the action of endorphins. The situation is still pretty confusing, but science thrives in uncertainty. Out of the morass of conflicting data will emerge new theories about the nature of mental illnesses, and more powerful and effective treatments for them.

In another brain-related area, endorphins may turn out to be connected with memory and learning. At least some experimental work with animals points at an involvement of endorphins with the ability to remember tasks learned via both positive and negative reinforcement. It is conceivable that someday we can make ourselves smarter or improve our memories by the use of endorphin injections or pills.

Still other possible endorphin connections exist—connections to the effects of alcohol on the brain; caffeine addiction; arthritis; anorexia nervosa; obesity; compulsive running; "runner's high"; the menstrual cycle; the functioning of our immune system; and the way we respond to and deal with different kinds of stress, including shock trauma.

Not only is this new wave in brain chemistry scientifically important; it will also surely prove to be economically important. Scientists already use genetic engineering techniques to make enough of these chemicals to use in the lab. The technology now exists to make them in huge quantities. Just as DNA-engineered bacteria can now make commercially available human insulin, and will soon make commercially available growth hormone and interferon, so it may only be a matter of a few years before endorphins will be available—perhaps by prescription, perhaps over the counter—in new medicines. If only a few of the possible endorphin connections prove positive, drug companies and genetic engineering firms will be most interested. And companies capable of producing in large quantities either synthetic or natural endorphins will be in a powerful market position.

* * *

The more we know about the brain, the less we know about the brain. The statement is paradoxical but true. The more we learn about the brain's workings, the more we realize how impossibly complex it is. And the more we come to appreciate that, the more some of us wonder about other kinds of questions. It is not just the physical and chemical structure of the brain that interests many people; it is the question of "the mind" and the brain. Are they one and the same? Are they different? Are we "ghosts in the machine," or is the machine all there is? Can our increasing understanding of the workings of brain chemicals like endorphins give us clues to the answer to that question?

More than this, even: we see the compartmentalization of science breaking down before our eyes. Pharmacology, biology, chemistry, medicine, philosophy and theology all intersect at the three-and-a-half-pound still point of the turning world. So, too, does the science of quantum physics, with its bizarre conception of reality itself as nothing more than a ghost created by ghosts. Where are endorphins in all this? If they are indeed chemicals which help power the brain and bring into it impressions of the "reality outside," then they must be involved in these questions, too.

As we move more deeply inward, we move more deeply outward. We know so much. We know so little. So much remains to know. Endorphins are the newest wave to break upon the shore of knowledge. What will the next one bring?

PART I

THE STAGE

1

The Wonder of Our Stage

The English writer Ben Jonson once called another English writer, William Shakespeare, "the applause, delight, the wonder of our stage." Those words could just as accurately have been applied to the Bard's brain. Or to ours. For the three-and-a-half-pound mass of tissue and fluid that sits behind our eyes and above our spines is indeed the wonder of the earthly stage on which we live. And the brain itself is a "wondrous stage" upon which is acted the intricate ballet called the human personality. This is a book about some of the "planks" of that "wondrous stage": certain chemicals in the brain that help to make us what and who we are. These chemicals are generally referred to as *endorphins*, and they've also been found in the intestines, stomach, adrenal glands, spinal cord and other parts of the body.

Endorphins are chemicals similar to heroin in their composition and operation. Two big differences are that they are dozens to hundreds of times more powerful than heroin; and endorphins are chemicals the human body manufactures for its own use. And not just the human body: endorphins were originally found in mice, cows and pigs, and have since been found in salmon, camels, chickens, toads and many other creatures.

These chemicals are almost certainly *neurotransmitters:* molecules that transmit information between and among the brain cells or *neurons.* Endorphins and other neurotransmitters help

link the one hundred-plus billion neurons of the human brain
together into an incredibly complex network: a living, thinking,
feeling, worshiping organ of flesh that sits in the bony cathedral
of the skull, atop a segmented bone column that itself contains
within it a cord of tissue that is an extension of the brain.

There are powerful and persuasive data to suggest that the
endorphins are also involved in much, much more than "just" the
operation of the brain. The fact that these chemicals are found in
so many other parts of the body is an indication of an extensive
repertoire.

Many different types of endorphins are currently known:
alpha-, beta- and gamma-endorphin; methionine- and leucine-
enkephalin; several dynorphins; and alpha- and beta-neo-endorphin. These are in turn parts of larger molecules called precursors. We're going to look at them all: at what they are, where
they come from; who discovered them and when, and how; and
what they may do on the wondrous stages of the brain and body.

A World of Chemicals and Molecules

In a very real sense, it can truly be said that the body is nothing
more than a gigantic complex of molecules and chemicals working together in harmony. Everything that exists is made of chemicals. That familiar television advertisement phrase—"Without
chemicals, *life* it*self* would be im*pos*sible!!"—is literally true, since
life itself can be defined as an extremely complex interaction of
certain kinds of chemicals. Biochemistry is the study of the chemical processes of biology. This book will have a lot to do with
biochemistry. It will have even more to do with neurobiology, the
study of how nerve cells store and recall information at the molecular level. And it will be about *neuropharmacology*, the study of
the operations of drugs and drug-like chemicals in the nervous
system.

Chemistry has a language, and it uses symbols for its basic
units, the atoms. Hydrogen is the simplest element or atom; its
symbol is *H*. Oxygen, about sixteen times heavier than hydrogen,

is *O*. Carbon is *C*. Gold is *Au*, because the ancient Latin word for gold was "*Au*rum." The element sodium is symbolized by *Na* (from "natrium," the ancient Latin word for sodium). Chlorine is *Cl*. A chemical compound familiar to all is formed from two atoms of hydrogen and one of oxygen. It's written as "H_2O." The "H_2" means there are two atoms of hydrogen in the compound—which of course is water. Another chemical compound is written as "CO_2." It has one carbon atom and two oxygen atoms. We call it carbon dioxide, with "dioxide" meaning two oxygen atoms attached.

Common table salt is "NaCl": an atom of sodium bound to one of chlorine. Salt is an object lesson in chemistry. Sodium is, by itself, a soft white solid element that burns violently in the presence of almost any oxygen, and thus in the air. Chlorine is a deadly poisonous gas. But combined together through the electromagnetic forces of their outer electron shells, sodium and chlorine make a harmless white crystal that, in proper quantities, is essential to life.

What on earth does all this have to do with the brain, and endorphins, and how and why we remember and feel pain and become heroin addicts? This: our bodies are chemical complexes, and our brains are electrochemical computers (of a sort). We're going to have to have at least a nodding acquaintance with chemical language to have some idea of what's going on.

The molecular compounds we're going to be concerned with are considerably more complex than water and salt and carbon dioxide. They're made of hundreds and thousands of atoms—in some cases, many tens of thousands of them. But things tend to group themselves in orders of complexity in nature, and each set of compounds can in turn be dealt with as a unit; each will have an embracing name and a language of symbols.

Let's take a look at some of these compounds.

Up the Life Ladder

First, life in general is made of chemical substances called *organic compounds*. They're called "organic" because they have carbon in them. Carbon, hydrogen and oxygen are the essential elements in organic compounds. They combine together in a delightfully beautiful dance of complexity to make prions, viruses, bacteria, sea slugs, chinook salmon, iridescent green frogs, swallowtail butterflies, gila monsters, the late *Tyrannosaurus rex*, scolding scrub jays, tree shrews, the late *Homo habilis* and my good friend Kerry Beaulieu. "It's all organic," as we used to say back in the sixties.

Next, there is a group of organic compounds called *amino acids*. Amino acids are marked by the presence of two chemical groups hanging on either end of the organic compound. On one end is an *amino group* (NH_2-), and on the other is a *carboxyl group* (-$COOH$). The basic chemical formula for an amino acid is "NH_2-R-$COOH$," where "R" is a particular kind of organic compound. Amino acids are the major building blocks of the physical chemical complex that is a living creature. About eighty amino acids occur in Nature, and twenty are essential to life. Some, the body produces; others must be gotten through food consumption. Just as chemical formulas are written out with the symbols for atoms, so the formulas for some more complicated compounds are written out using the abbreviations of the amino acids.

Amino acids are the building blocks of two very important types of organic molecules: peptides and proteins. A peptide is, briefly, a brief protein. An organic chemical compound made of only a few dozen or so amino acids is usually called a peptide. If it gets much bigger than that, it's called a protein. The smallest peptides we'll be examining are the enkephalins, with just five amino acids. They're sometimes called *pentapeptides* ("penta-" being the prefix meaning five) for that reason. The beta-endorphin peptide is made of thirty-one amino acids, and another one is thirty-two amino acids in length. All of these peptides are called *opioid* peptides. That's because they resemble in both structure and activity the class of chemicals called opiates. The most familiar opiates are the drugs morphine and heroin (which is refined from morphine). We'll find as we move through the history of the endorphins that they were really discovered in large part because of one man's interest in why chemicals like heroin and morphine do what they do to humans. That resemblance made it perfectly reasonable to call these newly discovered compounds "opioid peptides."

These chemicals are also often called *endogenous* opioid peptides. "Endogenous" simply means "inside." Endorphins are opiate chemicals made inside the body. Heroin and morphine are "exogenous" opiates, produced outside the body.

The endogenous opioid peptides known generically as endorphins are all parts of larger molecules called *precursors*. The precursors are proteins with tens of thousands of atoms combined in hundreds of amino acids.

The Code of Life

Two other large proteins are DNA, or deoxyribonucleic acid, and RNA (ribonucleic acid). They have a simple yet beautifully elegant structure: a double helix. That twisting ladder is the ladder of life. DNA (like RNA) is made of three parts: nitrogen-containing compounds called bases; a sugar; and a phosphate chemical. In DNA the sugar is a molecule called deoxyribose; the phosphate chemical is phosphoric acid; and the bases are four chemicals named adenine (A), guanine (G), thymine (T) and cytosine (C). Combined with the phosphoric acid, the four bases are called nucleotides. A, T, G, and C attach to each other only in certain ways, so they can form certain patterns or codes. A three-"letter" sequence of nucleotides is called a "codon." The codons are the instructions for amino acids, so a DNA molecule contains within it the information to make insulin, adrenalin, hemoglobin and all the other proteins and peptides that make up the body, including endorphins and their precursor proteins.

Hormones, the Chemical Messengers

We mentioned at the beginning that endorphins are found not only in the brain but also in other body tissues. That's pretty important. Endorphins are all definitely involved in the functioning of the central nervous system, the brain and the spinal cord, and are almost certainly neurotransmitters. But they are nevertheless found in other parts of the body that aren't involved in the cerebral processes of the brain. They are, for one certain instance, produced as part of the *endocrine system,* a collection of organs called glands which secrete compounds called hormones.

Hormones are chemicals, peptides or proteins, produced and released in one part of the body which tell other parts of the body to do something. They act at a distance from their points of origin. They get carried to their points of action by the bloodstream. Hormones have origin/action distances that can and are measured in centimeters and meters. There are chemicals produced in glands in the brain that act on tissues in our toes (for example, the growth hormone). Neurotransmitters and other neurochemicals, on the other hand, act at points extremely close to their places of origin. The distances are measured in thousandths and ten thousandths of a centimeter.

Some compounds seem to act both as hormones and as neurotransmitters. One example is a chemical called *epinephrine,* which is made in the adrenal glands, sitting on top of the kidneys down at the bottom of our backs. Epinephrine, sometimes called adrenalin, acts on the entire body. It speeds the heart up, restricts the blood vessels, relaxes the tiny tubes of the lungs and generally puts the entire body in a state of high alert. Thus epinephrine is a hormone; it acts at a distance. But it has also been found *in the brain,* where it seems to function as a neurotransmitter. Other neurotransmitters, including endorphins and enkephalins, have been found in the endocrine system functioning as hormones. So the picture of endorphins is not nearly as simple as it might first seem. Some scientists prefer to call both kinds of compounds "neuroregulators." Nature (clever lady!) has a way of using the same substances and structures over and over again in different ways, and that's what she seems to be doing with many chemicals in the body, including adrenalin—and endorphins.

The Organ with a Lot of Nerve(s)

At the beginning of this chapter we mentioned "the one hundred-plus billion neurons of the human brain." The brain is where a lot of the action is when it comes to endorphins. It's where some of the endorphins are created and operate. The brain is an organ of marvelous complexity and ofttimes subtle architecture. We'll take a closer look at it in Chapter 2. But before we look at the stage upon which endorphins play, let's learn a bit about its boards, the nerve cells.

Nerve cells, or *neurons,* are specialized cells in the body of any creature which *generate, integrate* and/or *conduct information.* The information is generated, integrated or conducted in the form of excited electrochemical states within and/or among the neurons. That excitation either is generated internally, inside the neuron, or arrives from the environment via so-called *affector cells.* The neurons then pass on the excited state/information to other neurons and eventually to *effector cells,* such as muscle cells.

Neurons don't *directly* make the creature do anything. They process information in a living system. The neuronal system is more complex than any other, because the processing of information is absolutely essential to anything else. Whether it be information about the outside world, or information about the internal state of the organism itself, the creature *must know* before it can act.

Neurons are made up of a cell body, or *perikaryon,* and one or more long *processes* or extensions. One is an *axon,* and there may be one or more *dendrites.*

The cell body can range in size from two to five hundred micrometers. A *micro-* of something is one millionth, so one micrometer is one millionth of a meter, or 0.0000394 inches. Sometimes the perikaryon's volume is equal to or more than that of the neuron's axon. But sometimes the axons and dendrites are extremely long or branched, and the cell body is a mere one ten-thousandth of the entire neuron. The cell body is made of protoplasm and has a complex structure. Near the center is the nucleus, where the cell's DNA is contained. The protoplasm outside the neuron's nucleus is called the *cytoplasm;* its outer "skin" is the cell membrane, and inside that, throughout the cytoplasm, are the other typical cell structures—microtubules, organelles, mitochondria, vacuoles, Golgi bodies and so forth.

The axon is the longest process of the neuron. In most nerve cells it transmits nerve impulses to the dendrites of the next neurons in line. The dendrites are shorter and more branched in structure than the axon. They function as "receivers." Axons can also transmit impulses to the cell body itself. Axons are bundled together to form *nerves*.

Neurons produce within themselves large amounts of protein to provide something akin to an internal "rapid transit system" called *axoplasmic transport*. Since the axons of some neurons can get to be very long, up to twenty-five centimeters (nearly ten inches), axoplasmic transport moves nutrients and other material from the cell body to the outermost points of the axon and dendrites, and then back again.

Neurons come in an astounding variety of shapes. The variety is not for variety's sake, though. Neurons are highly specialized, more so than other cells in the body. Pyramidal cells, Purkinje cells, basket neurons, Golgi cells of several kinds—all look different from the others and each has a different function in different parts of the brain.

Between the tip of one neuron's axon and the cell next to it is a gap, measured in microns, called a *synapse*. The neuron sending a signal across the synaptic gap is called the presynaptic neuron. The receiving neuron on the other side is the postsynaptic neuron. The synapse is where the action is, where neurotransmitter chemicals are released. And where some of the endorphins do their thing.

How the Neuron Works

Scientists group those fifty or more neurotransmitters and neurohormones into different families or systems, based on similarities of chemistry and action. They include the *cholinergic system* (remember: -ergic means energy), which has acetylcholine for its neurotransmitter; the *adrenergic,* with epinephrine and norepi-

nephrine (adrenalin and noradrenalin); the *dopaminergic*, with dopamine; *GABA-ergic*, with GABA (gamma-aminobutyric acid); *serotoninergic*, with serotonin; and several others. Each of these
systems has its own set of receptor sites on the brain neurons.
The most recently discovered neuroregulatory system in the central nervous system is the opiate system, with its opiate receptors.

Neurotransmitters are created inside the neuronal perikaryon,
in membrane-lined "bubbles" called *synaptic vesicles*. The vesicles
are moved from the perikaryon down the axon to the synaptic
region by axoplasmic transport. And there, at the membranous
"skin" of the axon's tip, the vesicles pop and the neurotransmitter is released into the synaptic gap. The whole process is electrochemical in nature, and after nearly a century of sustained scientific inquiry it is still not completely understood. But it seems to
work like this:

Each neuron, in its resting state, is electrically charged. It has a
negative polarization of about seventy millivolts relative to what's
beyond its outer membrane. The neuron achieves and keeps this
negative charge by means of "ion pumps" in the membrane. An
"ion" is an electrically charged atom. If it's missing one or more
electrons, it is positively charged, because the positive charge of
the protons at its center is dominant. If it has one or more extra
electrons, which are negatively charged particles, then the atom
is a negative ion. These ion pumps keep certain ions distributed
unequally across the cellular membrane. The atoms involved, for
the most part, are K+ and Na+ (positively charged potassium
and sodium), and Cl- (negatively charged chlorine).

When the nerve's membrane is disturbed, though, ions can
"leak across" in either direction. That will decrease the electrical
potential that exists across it. If the potential drops below a
certain level, another kind of electrical potential is created—an
action potential. It is a wave of electrical energy which streaks down
the neuron at about 125 meters per second (that's 410 feet per
second, or almost 280 miles per hour). When the impulse reaches
the synapse at the end of the axon, it causes the synaptic vesicles
to pop and release their load of neurotransmitters into the gap
between the axon tip and the next neuron (either its perikaryon
or one of its dendrites). Some neurotransmitters cause a decrease
in the electrical potential of the next neuron in line and move it
closer to firing. Other neurotransmitters are inhibitory and in-

hibit the neuron, making it less likely to fire and pass the impulse on. Meanwhile, the ion pumps in the first neuron's membrane have quickly (in a few thousandths of a second) reestablished the electrical charge of the neuron, and it's ready to be fired off again by the neuron behind *it*.

The neurotransmitters cause excitation or inhibition by fitting into and activating certain spots on the cell membrane called *receptor sites*. Receptor sites and neurotransmitter chemicals work much like locks and keys. The receptor is a bit like a three-dimensional lock, into which fits a three-dimensional neurotransmitter key. The key nestles into the "lock," opens it up and signals the neuron to change the polarization of its membrane.

There are many types of receptor sites on neurons, each sensitive to different kinds of neurotransmitters. Some receptors, though "officially" meant for one kind of neurotransmitter chemical, can be activated by high concentrations of others. They can also be unlocked by outside (exogenous) chemicals that have compositions and three-dimensional shapes that "fool" them into thinking they are being "talked to" by an honest-to-goodness neurotransmitter.

That's the simple explanation for how neurotransmission works via the receptor sites. There's more to it than just this, and we'll look in a bit more detail at receptor sites and at the action of a chemical called cAMP in Chapter 4.

Some Large Numbers

Each neuron has one axon, but that axon may well have a lot of little branches at its end sending signals to different locations. And each neuron, with several dendrites each having many branches, may have axons from dozens of other neurons feeding excitatory or inhibitory impulses onto both its dendrites and its central body. Thus each neuron can be the recipient of an intricate complex of interacting signals, all of them modifying, strengthening or inhibiting the signal that the neuron in turn will pass on to some other neuron down the line.

Tens upon tens of billions of them. All doing that to each other. Together. Simultaneously. Instant by instant, processing information from the inner and outer worlds, passing it on to the rest of the organism for its proper responses.

You and I are the organism in which this is happening, instant by instant. The organ that is doing all of this is the human brain.

We marvel at the speed and complexity of today's high-tech computers. And they are quite fast indeed. Electrons flow through the circuits at the speed of light, and nothing's faster than that. Compared to 300 million meters per second, the 125-meter-per-second speed of nerve impulses is practically a snail's crawl. Modern computers are also quite complex. A microchip smaller than a fingernail equals in computing power the whole of ENIAC, the room-sized monstrosity that ushered in the computer age in 1946.

But none of today's computers comes close in complexity to the human brain. The one-hundred-plus billion neurons that comprise our "biological computer" are each connected to an average of a thousand other neurons. An *average*. Some of the brain cells in the part of the brain called the cerebellum have connections with seventy thousand to a hundred thousand others. But at a minimum, we're talking about some *one hundred trillion* interconnections. A hundred trillion synapses, each similar to a simple on/off or yes/no switch. A hundred trillion yes/no pieces of information capable of being held in the human brain. That's a stupefyingly large number.

Only half of the human brain is devoted to what we like to call our "higher functions." Most of the rest of it is busy just keeping our body functioning. But even if many of our synapses are not in use, there are tens of trillions of them which are, and in various states of "yes/no" from moment to moment.

And that gives rise to another stupefyingly large number. As Dr. Carl Sagan pointed out in *The Dragons of Eden,* if the brain had just one synapse connecting two neurons, then it could exist in only one of two possible mental states—yes or no. If it had two synapses, it would have *four* potential mental states—yes and no, yes and yes, no and yes, or no and no. We'd write that mathematically as two to the second power, or 2^2; the "big 2" represents the two states of a synapse, yes or no; the exponent represents the number of synapses. Three synapses have eight possible states

(2^3). Four synapses, sixteen states (2^4); five, thirty-two states; and so on. If there are a hundred trillion synapses in the brain (a thousand synapses for each neuron) then *that* number is what we'd use for the exponent, and the number of possible states for the human brain is $2^{100,000,000,000,000}$. That's the number two multiplied by itself a hundred trillion times. There aren't even that many atoms in the known universe. But that's the potential of the human brain.

It's not surprising that humans are building computers, and not vice versa. The vice versa probably won't happen for a while.

This marvelous collection of brain cells and synapses, what's more, is not in some random arrangement. Four and a half billion years of evolution have produced an organ of astounding organization and complexity. Shakespeare said that "all the world's a stage" upon which we act. The brain is equally the stage upon which endorphins act, and upon which the new discoveries about those peptides even now take place.

2

A Peek
Inside the Works

The average human brain weighs about 1,400 grams, or a little over three pounds. It occupies a volume of around 1,400 cubic centimeters, or about 84 cubic inches. That's the size of a standard bowling ball, but less than a fifth of its weight. Within certain parameters, though, human brain size and weight have no correlation with human IQ. And there is a lot of variation in the figures. The heaviest human brain ever measured was 2,049 grams. No, it wasn't Einstein's (which was pretty close to the norm); it was the brain of a person with an idiot IQ. The famous French novelist Anatole France had a brain that weighed only 1,017 grams at his death. That's less than three quarters of the average. Jonathan Swift had a brain that weighed about 2,000 grams. The weight of the average human female brain is about 150 grams less than that of the average human male brain. Indeed, the weight and size of the human brain changes throughout life. The organ's weight triples between birth and adulthood, and then begins decreasing by about a gram per year.

Human brain weight and size have little to do with human IQ. But might they have any bearing on why *humans* are intelligent and other animals are not? Up to a point, yes. Animals smaller than us have brains that are smaller than the human one, and with the possible exception of chimpanzees (who have brains that in size and weight are similar to those of human children and some genetically retarded humans with small brains) none are blessed with intelligence. On the other hand, there are a number of animals larger than us, with larger brains, and no real evidence that they are also intelligent. That characteristic has been imputed to elephants, dolphins and whales, all with brains larger than ours; but so far no one's come up with good, clean, hard evidence to prove the contention.

Some people contend that what's important is the brain-to-body weight ratio. The weight of a human brain is 2.5 percent of the body's weight. The closer the percentage for an animal is to the human, the argument goes, the more likely that the animal might be intelligent, or capable of being so. This, of course, would explain why whales and elephants may possess brains larger than ours but are nonetheless not intelligent. The elephant's brain weight is only 0.2 percent of its body weight. For the whale the figure is 0.003 percent. For dogs it's 0.85 percent. For rats, 0.48 percent. On the other hand, in both the sparrow (4.2 percent) and the spider monkey (4.8 percent) the percentage is larger than in humans, and no one's ever accused either creature of tendencies toward cubism, haute cuisine or controlled thermonuclear war. The answer to this particular question lies not in the gross characteristics of size and weight, but in the brain's architecture and internal structure. So let's take a peek inside the works.

From the Top

The brain consists of three sections: the *forebrain,* the *midbrain* and the *hindbrain.* Most of the forebrain is the two cerebral hemispheres, or the cerebrum. The midbrain is basically the top part of the brainstem. The hindbrain is the rest of the brainstem plus the structure called the cerebellum. The brain itself is part of the *central nervous system* (CNS), which also includes the brainstem and the spinal cord. The *peripheral nervous system* is not structurally separate from the CNS, but is spoken of separately because its function is different. It supplies information from the outside world to the CNS and ultimately the brain. The CNS processes that data and makes decisions based on it.

(An American scientist named Paul McLean has suggested that the brain can be divided into three parts on the basis of evolutionary development. In his scheme, the cerebrum is the "new mammalian brain," the part of the forebrain known as the limbic system is the "old mammalian brain," and the midbrain and hindbrain are called "the reptilian brain." It's a neat-sounding description, and there's considerable truth to it. It is also a touch oversimplified.)

To get at the human brain we remove the top of the skull, slice through three thin layers of tissue—and there it is: a mass of living matter about the size of a ripe cantaloupe, the consistency of cooked oatmeal and the color of good Pacific Northwest pink salmon. Yes, this is the "gray matter"—but it's gray only when the brain is dead and sitting in preserving fluid. The color of a normal, healthy living brain is pinkish-brown. Its surface is quite wrinkled.

The brain gets its nutrients and oxygen through the circulatory system. The *neuroglia* transfers nutrients and oxygen from the blood to the neurons. The neuroglia is non-nervous tissue in the brain which also functions as "insulation" for the neurons. In addition, it is part of the *blood-brain barrier* (BBB), which lets some substances in (many drugs get across) but screens almost everything else out, including chemicals made in some glands within the brain.

We are looking at the *cerebrum,* which makes up fully 70 percent of the brain proper. It is part of the forebrain, and its upper surface is called the *neocortex.* The cerebrum, or "cerebral cortex," is where all our sensory experiences, all that massive amount of data from the "outside world," are mixed and blended together into what we call reality.

The cerebrum's convolutions increase its surface area. Were it billiard-ball smooth, the cortex would have a surface area of about 60,000 square millimeters. But the wrinkles give it an effective area of more than 200,000 square millimeters, or 324 square inches. *Why* does the human brain have so much surface area? Even though it increases the brain's total volume by only a little, it more than triples its total surface area. From an area equal to that of a sheet of standard-sized notebook paper, it increases to that of a chessboard eighteen inches on a side. On that board is played out the intricate game of human intelligence.

Our highly wrinkled cerebral cortex sets us apart from most other animals, who have brains with relatively few folds. Some have hardly any cerebral cortex to *have* folds. So while the spider monkey and sparrow may have brain-to-body ratios better than ours, they have nothing in the way of convoluted cerebral cortexes. The same goes for dogs and rats. Whales and dolphins do have brains nearly as convoluted as ours, and certainly (in the case of whales) more massive.

Is there, then, an intelligence/brain-wrinkle connection? It's never been proven. Lots of people think whales and dolphins are intelligent. Lots of other people *want* whales and dolphins to be intelligent. Believing it, wanting it—these are not nearly the same as *proving* it. Turing's principle of artificial computer intelligence applies here: you're locked in a room and you are communicating with an entity beyond the room through a teletypewriter; if the responses you're getting are indistinguishable from a human's, then the entity you are talking with has human intelligence—even if it is a computer. No computer has yet passed that test. Neither have whales or dolphins or elephants or chimps.

The neocortex, the uppermost part of the cerebrum, is just 4.5 millimeters thick, about the height of a typewritten letter "l". And some estimates have more than eight billion neurons in the neocortex alone.

Though incredibly thin, the neocortex has six distinct layers. They are called the molecular layer, the external granular layer, the outer pyramidal layer, the internal granular layer, the ganglionic layer and the multiform layer. They are in turn made of billions of highly specialized neurons with names like granule cells, Martinotti cells, pyramidal cells, stellate cells, and so on. All are arranged in an intricate order. The main body of a neuron may be in one layer, but may have an axon extending up or down through several others. The complexity here is more than astounding. There are something like ten thousand *miles* of interconnecting nerve tissue in each cubic *inch* of neocortex. That's enough connections to stretch from Los Angeles to Cape Town and back twenty-eight times. Enough to stretch from here to the moon and back again, and then back to the moon *again*.

Below the thin layer of the neocortex is the white matter. We can't see it yet, but we will soon enough. Then we'll use microscopes and we'll notice that here, too, hundreds of millions of neurons are interconnected in a marvelously complex manner.

The next thing we do notice, almost immediately, is that the cerebral cortex is bilateral in structure. It has two distinct sides. We conveniently label them the left and right hemispheres. Dividing the two hemispheres from each other is a space called the *longitudinal fissure*.

If we look more closely, we may also discern other divisions and other fissures. Those divisions are called the brain's *lobes*. At the front of the brain are the two *frontal* lobes. Behind them are the *parietal* lobes, separated from the frontal lobes by the *Rolandic* (or central) fissure. The parietal lobes run across the top of the head and toward the back. At the sides of the head, in the region of our ears and temples, are the two *temporal* lobes. The *Sylvian* fissures separate them from the frontal and parietal lobes. Finally, at the rear of the brain and not separated from anything by any fissure, are the two *occipital* lobes.

The two hemispheres have come in for a lot of publicity in the last few years. Many books have touted the differences in function between the two hemispheres. The "left brain," they claim, specializes in language ability and is logical, linear, mathematical, rigid and structured; the "right brain" determines spatial perception and is intuitive, holistic, creative, mystical and generally mellow.

The left-brain/right-brain dichotomy has been much overplayed. The right hemisphere controls the left side of the body, and vice versa. But the business of intelligence and creativity is not quite so specialized. It is possible to track the brain's activity by monitoring the flow of blood which has been tagged with a mild radioactive tracer. The more active a part of the brain, the more blood flows through it, and the more intense is the reading from the radioactive tracer. When some volunteers for such a test were asked to speak aloud, more blood entered their left hemispheres—but their right hemispheres also received a surge. When they were asked to perform tasks that involved manipulating spatial concepts, the right hemisphere lit up. And so did the left, though the right was dominant. The point is that both hemispheres work together, and there is no real exclusivity when it comes to these kinds of functions. It's share and share (almost) alike.

Years of experimentation with humans undergoing brain surgery, as well as observations of people with certain kinds of brain damage (what some have called "nature's experiments"), have led us to discover different functions controlled in different parts of the cerebrum. For example, in the mid- and late nineteenth century Sir David Ferrier mapped a part of the cerebrum that's called the *motor cortex,* and discovered another part called the *sensory strip.* Each hemisphere has a motor cortex, a strip of brain tissue that initiates muscular activity. In front of the motor cortex is another strip called the premotor cortex, which controls and plans movement begun by the motor cortex. The motor cortex has many discrete regions controlling separate and distinct actions. A large amount of motor cortex is devoted simply to initiating and controlling the action of our hands and our lips.

The sensory strip or cortex lies near the motor cortex. Each hemisphere has one. It receives and deals with the sensations arriving from different body parts. Again, a relatively large area of the sensory strip is devoted to data coming from our hands and face. It should be no surprise that this is the case for both the motor and sensory cortexes. So much of what makes us distinctively human has to do with our hands and face and lips and mouths. We do so much of our communicating that way; we interact in subtle and profound ways with our world through our hands and face. We are the toolmakers; the talkers; the laughers.

Speaking of speaking: in 1861 a French scientist named Paul Broca identified a location in the left cerebral hemisphere which is associated with speech. It's now called Broca's area, and it controls speech *production.* Another part of the brain is also involved in speech. It was first identified by Carl Wernicke in 1874, and it is called (are we surprised?) Wernicke's area. It's located in the left temporal and parietal lobes, and it controls the *understanding* of speech. Curious, that: production and understanding are separate functions related to speech; they are not the same, and different parts of the brain control them. And the specialization gets even more detailed. One part of Wernicke's area, for instance, deals with naming things; another part with repetition of spoken words. If still another part of the area is damaged, the person cannot read pictographic script like Chinese writing, but can read English, which is phonetic.

But even this explanation is an oversimplification. Other parts of the brain are also involved in understanding and making language. If we electrically disrupt the parts of the motor strip that control the sequence of mouth movements that make speech sounds, we find the person not only can't make those sounds but can't recognize them upon hearing them. Localization of speech and language differs from person to person. Only the areas of the motor strip that relate to speech stay constant.

There's much, much more to learn about the cerebrum, more than we have time or room for in this book. We will, though, come back in a bit and look at the interior of the forebrain, the areas deep in the brain that are old and primitive and essential to life itself. First, though, let's go on and look at the midbrain and hindbrain.

A Look at the Midbrain

The *midbrain,* also called the "mesencephalon," is a small structure (about 2.5 centimeters, or less than an inch) that sits atop the brainstem, which in turn sits atop the spinal column. The midbrain governs some of our reflex muscle actions, such as the movements made by the pupils of our eyes. Here also is the *reticular formation,* a group of nerves and fibers in a diffuse formation filling nooks and crannies throughout the brainstem. The reticular formation helps to control waking, sleeping and various reflexes. It warns our forebrain if it's necessary to move from sleep consciousness to wakeful-state consciousness.

The third and fourth pairs of cranial nerves, sensory nerves which serve our eye muscles, pass through the midbrain. A nerve pathway from the tectum, or "roof," of the midbrain, called the *superior colliculus,* helps coordinate visual data with posture. It's one reason we don't fall flat on our faces every time we try to stand up. This pathway is also involved with the function of feature extraction, essential for knowing what we're looking at.

Here, too, is a small nucleus of neurons called the *substantia nigra* which is extremely important in the governing of movement and muscular control. The substantia nigra is the major producer of the neurotransmitter *dopamine* (sometimes abbreviated as DA). If for some reason the substantia nigra does not produce enough DA, the person will suffer from Parkinson's disease, characterized by slowness and loss of movement, muscular rigidity, a peculiar stooped stance, and tremors in the muscles that can often spread throughout the body. Once incurable, Parkinson's disease can now be treated with doses of a chemical called L-dopa, which the brain can convert to dopamine.

Other structures in the midbrain, and their functions, include:

• the *inferior colliculus,* which helps with the correlation of information about sound sources, equilibrium, the displacement of images underwater, localization of other sensory inputs and in some animals the detection of electrical fields.

• the *periaqueductal gray matter,* or PAG, which is an extremely important part of the limbic system and its associated control of emotions.

• the *red nucleus,* which is involved in motor coordination. It's not well developed in primates (we're primates), but is in carnivorous animals—lions, tigers and suchlike, which certainly need a well-developed sense of motor coordination.

Down to the Bottom

The hindbrain, or brainstem, sits below the midbrain and the forebrain and above the spinal cord, which actually runs down from the hindbrain. It consists of the *medulla oblongata,* the *pons* and the *cerebellum.*

The cerebral cortex gets all the glory, because that's where intelligence and self-awareness are thought to rest. But the cerebellum, medulla and brainstem are also vitally important.

The cerebellum lies at the back of the brain and is about the size of a ripe plum. It's made up of a multitude of neurons grouped into many thin, fold-like structures which are arranged in two large masses flanking a middle portion. It has a huge number of connections with the cerebrum above and the spinal cord below. The cerebellum is like a switchboard; it coordinates different complex movements into specialized actions. Example: I'm sitting here at my word processor, typing these words. As I do it, I glance at my notes. Then I look at the screen to see what I'm typing, noticing miscues and backing the cursor up to erase them and make corrections. Meanwhile, my fingers fly on the keys. And all the time the radio is going in the background, playing some Latin jazz that goes just fine with an afternoon that's been pretty jazzy so far.

These are all complex movements that I'm making. Many different muscles in fingers, wrists, forearms, eyes, neck and shoulders are moving. They are in turn being influenced by what my eyes see and, to a lesser extent, by the bouncy music in the background. The cerebellum is the part of my brain that is doing that coordinating. Without it, I'd be totally helpless. I'd certainly have trouble doing the simplest tasks, with no ability to coordinate the movements of my muscles.

In front of the cerebellum, and right on top of the spinal cord, is the *medulla oblongata*. It's about two and a half centimeters (one inch) long. For such a tiny piece of nerve tissue, the medulla is essential to life. Cell concentrations in the medulla control our breathing, heartbeat, swallowing, digestion and metabolism. Also in the medulla, nerves from the two cerebral hemispheres cross and head down into the spine. Thus the right hemisphere controls the left side of our bodies, and vice versa.

Lying just above the medulla, and essentially a part of it, is the *pons*. The pons is made of massive nerve fiber bundles that begin in the cerebrum and move back into the cerebellum. Thus the pons takes part in the coordination of hearing, sight, movement and various sensations.

These different brain sections (forebrain/cerebrum, midbrain, hindbrain/cerebellum, pons, medulla) are all pretty much visible to us as we gaze on the human brain. Hidden inside, though, underneath the cerebral cortex and above the medulla and pons, are several other structures that are part of the forebrain but act in a sense as "between-brain" centers (and are technically referred to as the *diencephalon,* or "between-brain"). They are key locations in our quest for endorphins.

So we do some cutting and slicing. (We're not working on a live human brain now, but one from a cadaver.) Now we see the white matter of the inner cerebrum. If we look at a slice under a microscope we will see how the brain cells of the cortex are arranged in columns—millions of them, with hundreds of millions of interconnections.

We cut deeper; more slices; we separate the two hemispheres by cutting the *corpus callosum*, the massive connecting band of nerves that integrates the two hemispheres. We continue; we find spaces in the brain. These are the ventricles, once thought to contain "animal spirits" but shown by the Italian anatomist Domenico Cotugno in 1774 to contain only cerebrospinal fluid.

We press onward; and we find the limbic system, which helps modulate joy and hate, love and sorrow, all our emotion and also our memory (for how can we get emotional about something if we cannot remember it?). Here are the left and right thalamus, the hippocampus, the fornix, the mammillary body; the two cingulate gyri, the olfactory bulb, the amygdala.

And finally we come to it: the "between-brain" structures of the diencephalon. The first one we want to look at is the *pituitary gland*. It is part of the body's endocrine system and is about the size and weight of a pea. The pituitary sits at the base of the brain, right behind one of the skull's sinus cavities. It's joined to the brain by a stalk of tissue that extends down from the floor of one of the ventricles.

The pituitary is divided into anterior and posterior lobes. It also has a tiny section called the intermediate lobe. Some fifty thousand nerve fibers descend from the brain into the pituitary gland, which also has an extensive blood supply. Obviously, the pituitary is a very important gland. In fact, the pituitary's been called the body's master gland, because so many hormones are made there.

Hormones that are made or released from the anterior lobe include *growth hormone;* ACTH; and *thyrotropin,* or TTH, which regulates our thyroid glands. Here, too, are released the hormones regulating our reproductive systems: *follicle-stimulating hormone* (FSH), which stimulates the development of eggs in women and sperm in men; *luteinizing hormone,* or LH, which along with FSH governs the release of estrogen and ovulation in women;

and *prolactin*, which governs the release of progesterone and induces the secretion of milk in developed mammary glands.

Some of the hormones made in the pituitary and other glands of the endocrine system also appear in the brain as neurotransmitters. However, they usually don't move from those glands into the brain. (The blood-brain barrier, a membrane which lines the capillaries in the brain, keeps them out.) Rather, they are made by the neurons that use them. This is true of chemicals such as epinephrine (adrenalin), norepinephrine (noradrenalin) and dopamine, among others. It's just one of many cases of nature doing double duty with the same compounds.

Hormones don't seem to be made in the posterior lobe of the pituitary. Rather, hormones made in another gland called the *hypothalamus* are released through the posterior lobe. They include *oxytocin*, which acts on the uterus, and *vasopressin*, which induces contraction of blood vessels and also helps to prevent excessive loss of water through the kidneys.

The hypothalamus, where oxytocin and vasopressin are made, is extremely important. If the pituitary is the body's master gland, then the hypothalamus is the overlord. Indeed, we could rightly call the pituitary an extension of the hypothalamus, for the latter controls the release of hormones from the former. Regulation of our heartbeat rate, body temperature, metabolism, processing of water and fat, sexual development, and sleep—all are ultimately governed by the hypothalamus. In large part that's because it is the site where *hormone-releasing factors* are created.

These factors trigger the formation of the hormones released by the pituitary and other endocrine glands. Here in the hypothalamus are created LHRH, the luteinizing-hormone *releasing* hormone; TRH, the thyrotropin *releasing* hormone; GHRH, the gonadotropic-hormone *releasing* hormone (which governs FSH); and others. Some of those others include huge molecules that are broken down in the pituitary gland's posterior lobe to produce a class of peptide chemicals discovered less than ten years ago: endorphins.

3

The Discovery
of Endorphins

Where does the discovery of endorphins really begin? As with
any scientific discovery, there really is no specific beginning. Everything is connected to everything else. Discoveries made today
depend on the work done last year or in the last century. So the
discovery of endorphins can be said to begin with Otto Loewi's
discovery in 1921 that acetylcholine is a neurotransmitter; or with
Santiago Ramón y Cajal's theory of synaptic transmission of information among nerves, in 1901; or with Charles Brown-Sé-
quard's nineteenth-century work on the endocrine system. We
can even go back to the sixth century B.C., and to Pythagoras, who
declared that the brain was the organ of the mind. In many ways
the discovery of endorphins is connected to all these. But most
immediately, the discovery of endorphins began twenty years ago
in San Francisco, with a protein discovered by a biochemist from
Canton, China.

Carving the Pituitary

Choh Hao Li, a professor of biochemistry and experimental endocrinology, is head of the Hormone Research Laboratory at the

University of California, San Francisco. A distinguished-looking man, Li was born in Canton, China, and came to the United States in 1935. He has worked at the Hormone Research Laboratory at UCSF since 1950.

In 1964, Li and his colleagues were working on ACTH, a vitally important hormone. ACTH (which stands for *adrenocortico-tropic hormone*) is produced in the pituitary gland in the brain and from there travels to the adrenal glands lying on top of the kidneys. There it acts to regulate the release of adrenal hormones like norepinephrine, which acts as a vasoconstrictor, causing the blood vessels to narrow in width.

Li and his associates had been at the forefront of the work that eventually isolated ACTH and determined its chemical structure. They had been the first to make synthetic ACTH that was biologically active. They were also busy making synthetic versions of parts of the ACTH molecule, to see which parts were the ones that gave ACTH its potency.

Chemicals like ACTH are never present in very large amounts, so the people who work with these substances are always looking for ways to produce more from a given supply of pituitary glands (which usually come from slaughtered cattle, sheep or pigs). Li and his lab assistants had come up with a way of doing that. Part of the new technique involved different ways of cutting up the pituitary glands. The stuff that came out of the specially carved pituitaries had to be purified, of course, to get pure ACTH to work on. And it was while they were analyzing the substances obtained during their new carving techniques that Li came across a new compound in the pituitary. Something that was not ACTH.

It was a new protein. And it was pretty tiny. The first results indicated it had a molecular weight of about sixty nine hundred daltons. A "dalton" is a measurement of mass equal to about six ten-trillionths of a trillionth of a trillionth of an ounce. (If you prefer the metric system, it's about 1.6 hundred-billionths of a trillionth of a trillionth of a gram.) Even sixty-nine hundred daltons is not much. The chemical appeared to be made of fifty-nine amino acids, those chemical building blocks of all living things, and it showed weak lipolytic activity—it was stimulating lipid or fat-producing cells. So Li named the protein "lipotropin," from Greek words meaning "fat" and "turning" or "stimulating."

The first published report about lipotropin appeared in February 1964. Late in 1965, Li and Livio Barnafi, Michel Chrétien and David Chung announced they had figured out the actual amino acid structure of a version of lipotropin found in sheep pituitary glands called *beta-lipotropin,* or beta-LPH. While the sequence of amino acids they published was not entirely accurate, it was very close. Beta-LPH turned out to have ninety-one amino acids, not fifty-nine, and it weighed about ten thousand daltons, not six thousand.

The discovery of beta-lipotropin didn't raise many waves in the scientific world. The only really interesting thing about it was that it had embedded in it the entire amino acid sequence for one other pituitary-made protein, and part of a second. The amino acid sequence in beta-LPH from forty-one to fifty-eight was also the complete amino acid sequence for a protein called *beta-melanocyte-stimulating hormone,* or beta-MSH. This is the hormone that stimulates skin cells to form melanin, the skin-coloring agent. Beta-lipotropin also contained part of the amino acid sequence of ACTH. But that was it. Nothing else seemed to be going on with beta-lipotropin.

C. H. Li was still interested in his new protein. He wondered about the similarities and differences in the beta-LPH of different animals. Such comparisons could well give clues to how the species evolved over time. Li had many other things to work on that were more pressing. However, he also had a research fellow working for him who was from Iraq. Li figured that Iraq and neighboring Iran had lots of camels. Camels were lean beasts, unlike pigs and cows. It would be interesting to find out if the beta-LPH produced by their pituitary glands was the same as bovine and porcine beta-LPH. He asked his associate to gather some camel pituitary glands when he got back home.

It took two years to get five hundred camel pituitary glands, barely enough to mash and blend and strain and process in order to gather enough beta-LPH to test. And he did get some interesting answers to the question of differences among the beta-LPH of different species. But basically the beta-lipotropin sat on the shelf for nearly a decade.

Then in 1971 something happened to pull it off the shelf and into the limelight.

A Tie That Binds

Everyone involved in the study of opiate drugs such as morphine and heroin had assumed for some time that those substances acted in the brain; and that the reason they acted in the brain was that the brain neurons had receptor sites for them. The question was: Why? Why should the human brain have evolved receptor sites for heroin? What conceivable pro-survival use would such a development have? There was simply no reason for the brain to have such sites.

Unless, of course, the receptors (or binding sites, as they're often called) were *not* for heroin. Unless the brain was producing chemicals *similar in structure* to morphine and heroin; producing them in some unknown location for some unknown purpose. If the brain was actually doing this, then it would need receptors on its neurons for these homegrown chemicals to plug into. And if heroin and morphine were similar to these brain-produced chemicals, then they'd fool neuronal receptors when they entered the brain.

The hypothesis made sense. The problem was that (1) no one had ever found such receptor sites, and (2) no one had ever found opiate-like chemicals produced in the brain.

Enter Avram Goldstein, head of the Addiction Research Foundation in Palo Alto, California, and a professor of pharmacology at Stanford University. Born in New York City in 1919, he has A.B. and M.D. degrees from Harvard, and is one of the world leaders in research on opiate drugs and narcotic addiction. He's authored or coauthored hundreds of research papers, and several books that are standard texts in the field of pharmacology. He is also very tall and looks a bit like Aleksandr Solzhenitsyn, winner of the 1970 Nobel Prize for Literature. This resemblance will no doubt be commented on if (more likely, when) Goldstein gets one for medicine.

In August 1971, Goldstein suggested some new and specific ways to look for such "opiate receptors" in the brain. The method involved a condition called stereoisomerism, in which two substances may have identical chemical formulas but are also mirror images of each other. One is "left-handed" and the other is "right-handed." Goldstein showed how it might be possible to use opiates which were stereoisomers to show the existence and location of their receptor sites. In fact, in the process of developing his method he came up with a result in mouse brain tissue that he thought might have been caused by the still theoretical opiate receptor sites. That inspired a lot of people to go and look for them. They included Eric Simon of the New York University School of Medicine; Lars Terenius of Uppsala University in Sweden; and two people at Johns Hopkins University Medical School, Solomon Snyder and his graduate assistant Candace Pert. All three hit pay dirt at almost the same time. Pert and Snyder's journey to discovery is illustrative.

Candace Pert was a twenty-four-year-old graduate student in 1972. Two years earlier she had been inspired to go into the field of brain research after hearing a talk by Nobel Prize winner Gerald Nirenberg, who had switched his field of research from DNA to brain cells. Later, she is reported to have said, she was getting injections of morphine for a broken back and came across some of Goldstein's papers dealing with the possible existence of opiate receptors. She decided to try and begin research with her mentor in that area.

Her mentor was Solomon Snyder, a professor of psychiatry and pharmacology at Johns Hopkins. Born in 1938, Snyder got his M.D. at Georgetown University in 1962. He's been probing the mysteries of drugs and drug interactions throughout his professional life, and—like Goldstein—is an acknowledged expert in the field. He's also an expert in classical guitar.

In a series of experiments in 1972, the two Johns Hopkins researchers looked for the theoretical opiate receptors in the brains of mice. As part of the process they used small amounts of radioactively tagged *naloxone*. Naloxone is a chemical known to counteract the effects of opiate drugs like morphine. It is sometimes used to treat people who had overdosed on heroin. The theory was that naloxone blocked the effect of the opiates by filling up the receptor sites and preventing the opiates from "plugging into" them. Snyder and Pert also figured that, if this were true, so was the opposite: if the opiates were introduced first, they would plug into the receptor sites and prevent naloxone from filling them.

The two researchers added the naloxone to a mixture of homogenized mouse brain and special fluid buffers, and filtered the mixture. Then they used a scintillation counter (similar to a Geiger counter) to determine how much of the radioactively tagged naloxone had actually been "bound up" in the homogenized brain tissue.

When Pert and Snyder first added opiates like methadone or morphine to the mashed mouse brains, they found that very little of the naloxone stayed in. It did not bind very well. Indeed, the more powerful the opiate drug they used, the more it blocked the binding of the naloxone.

But when they first added *non-opiate* drugs or chemicals like serotonin or norepinephrine to the brain mixture, the naloxone remained in higher quantities. That meant it was *opiate-type* chemicals that were involved in this binding activity, and not just brain chemicals in general.

Snyder and Pert thus showed that opiate drugs were indeed binding to sites in the brain, preventing the radioactively tagged naloxone from plugging in. The brain cells (at least, of mice) definitely did have binding or receptor sites for opiates. It was theory no longer. They were well and truly there.

The two Johns Hopkins researchers also found the radioactively tagged naloxone was binding to opiate receptors in guinea pig intestines. That suggested that they were on the right track, since guinea pig intestinal tissue was often used to test for the presence and strength of opiate narcotics. It made perfect sense that they'd find them there.

Now brain researchers *really* got interested. Almost certainly there was a still undiscovered chemical lurking in the brain. Something *like* morphine, or heroin, or methadone. An "endogenous" ("from the inside") opiate-like chemical made in the brain and intestines. If it were there—well, the implications were enormous. It might explain the physical mechanism of drug addiction; and why some people become insane and how some drugs help them (and some don't); and how and why we feel pain.

The Race

Pert and Snyder were not the only ones to find evidence of opiate receptors in the brain; Eric Simon and Lars Terenius had also found them. As is often the case in science, several people were working on the same problem, and several people found the same answer at practically the same time. Now, though, the race was on to find the chemical or chemicals in the brain that the opiate receptors were there to receive.

And it *was* a race. The people involved understood the implications. They knew what it might mean to find chemicals in the brain that were like heroin. They were human, they liked being first, and they liked being recognized as being first. It was important to be respected by their peers. And if perchance they got awards, all the better. Should a Nobel Prize come one's way, fine. What was important about the Nobel was that it was a sign of recognition by one's peers.

The scientific teams in the race to find the endogenous opioids included Avram Goldstein and his group at Stanford University; John Hughes, Hans Kosterlitz and their associates in Scotland; Lars Terenius at the University of Uppsala; Eric Simon at NYU; and Roger Guillemin, Nicholas Ling and Richard Burgus at the Salk Institute in San Diego, California.

Almost everyone in the search found them, and nearly simultaneously. If one goes by the date of publication of papers reporting discoveries, then Lars Terenius gets the laurels for first finding the searched-for chemicals. But in a not uncommon twist of scientific fate, Terenius's paper seems to have been forgotten, or at least not considered precise enough for first-place credit. Instead, it was John Hughes who got credit for hitting pay dirt first. On May 2, 1975, he announced the discovery of a substance extracted from the ubiquitous blended mixture of small mammal brains. In this case it was some guinea pigs, rabbits, rats and pigs that gave their all for science.

John Hughes was a young (born on the Feast of the Three Kings in 1942, he was just thirty-three at the time) and good-looking fellow who got his B.A. at Chelsea College, London, and his Ph.D. at the Institute of Basic Medical Sciences. He began working at the University of Aberdeen in Scotland in 1969, work-

ing both on his own and under the mentorship of Dr. Hans
Kosterlitz.

Hughes and the Scottish team at the University of Aberdeen
found a substance of "low molecular weight" which "inhibits
neurally evoked contractions of the mouse vas deferens and
guinea pig myenteric plexus." By "low molecular weight" they
meant a substance that weighed around seven hundred daltons,
or perhaps a bit more. That's a lot less than the ten thousand
daltons of beta-lipotropin, for example. So the Hughes compound was a very small one.

There was no doubt that the substance they found was endogenous, or produced in the brain. But how did they know that it
plugged into the morphine receptor found by Pert and Snyder?
The answer to that is in the mouse vas deferens and the guinea
pig myenteric plexus. So at the risk of getting a bit over-medical,
let's take a quick look at them.

The *vas deferens* is the little tube that carries sperm from the
testes of the male mammal. It connects to the urethra, the tube
that in the male mammal carries sperm or urine to its discharge
point at the end of the penis. The *myenteric plexus* is a network of
blood vessels and nerves in the muscular lining of the intestine.
The phrase comes from Latin and Greek: plexus from a Latin
word meaning "network," itself from an earlier Latin word meaning "to plait" or "to braid"; and myenteric from two Greek words
—*mys*, meaning "muscle," and *enteron*, meaning "intestine."

A standard way of testing the strength of opiate drugs is to
observe the way they affect portions of an animal's intestine.
Usually it's guinea pig myenteric plexus that's used. The mouse
vas deferens is also good for this. Researchers will stimulate the
tissue electrically by attaching small electrodes to it. Then they
will place some of the opiate substance to be tested on the vas
deferens and/or the myenteric plexus, and again electrically
stimulate it. The effect of the opiate is to inhibit the reaction of
the tissue to the electrical stimulation. There's a direct correlation between the strength of the opiate compound and its ability
to inhibit the stimulation of the vas deferens and/or myenteric
plexus.

Hughes and his colleagues took the brains of rabbits, guinea
pigs, rats and pigs, and subjected them to a long process of
freezing, powdering, filtering and extracting. At the end of the

process they found a previously unknown substance. Pert and
Snyder had already shown that the opiate receptors they discovered were not only present in the brains of rats and guinea pigs,
but also in other areas—including the mouse vas deferens and
the guinea pig myenteric plexus. Hughes knew all this, and what
he showed was that his newly discovered brain chemical *affected
the vas deferens the same way morphine did.* Just as importantly, the
"opiate antagonist" naloxone *counteracted his new chemical the same
way it did morphine.*

These results were not one-shot things. They were typical of
forty-two consecutive experiments. Other substances did inhibit
the vas deferens twitch; dopamine, for example, and norepinephrine and a couple of prostaglandin substances. They are all hormones or neurotransmitters found in the brain. Naloxone did not
counteract their inhibitory effects, as it did both the newly discovered brain compound and morphine. Nearly a dozen other brain
chemicals tested on the mouse vas deferens did not inhibit its
contractions. And the naloxone by itself did not inhibit the
twitch, either.

Thus Hughes showed that the brain chemical he had extracted
was not a previously known brain chemical that either did or did
not have an effect in the mouse vas deferens opiate test; that the
chemical itself did have an effect similar to exogenous opiates like
morphine; that his new chemical was itself affected by naloxone,
as were exogenous opiates; and that it wasn't naloxone that was
inhibiting the twitches of the vas deferens, but the new chemical
he had discovered.

It was a beautifully elegant piece of work, with all bases cov-
ered, all holes plugged. There was no escaping the home run
conclusion:

John Hughes had found the first known endogenous opiate.

He named it *enkephalin,* from *en-,* "in," and *cephalo-,* "head."

Grand Slam

Everyone else was right behind him.

The scene broke open at a conference sponsored by the International Narcotic Research Club, at Airlie House, Virginia, on May 21–24, 1975:

• Hughes and three associates (Terry Smith, Barry Morgan and Linda Fothergill) presented a paper on their continuing work with enkephalin.

• Lars Terenius and Agneta Wahlstrom also announced their discovery of a chemical that seemed identical to the enkephalin of Hughes et al. They were calling it a "morphine-like substance" or factor (MLF).

• Solomon Snyder, Gavril Pasternak and Robert Goodman had also found enkephalin-type compounds in their series of experiments.

All three teams agreed that the compound had a molecular weight of about one thousand daltons; that it was definitely interacting with morphine receptors in brain and intestinal tissues; that its effect was counteracted by morphine antagonists like naloxone; and that it was considerably more powerful than morphine.

At the same conference Avram Goldstein and his team had two papers that dealt with the isolation, purification and properties of two peptide-like substances from pituitaries taken from commercially slaughtered cattle. They were similar in some ways to enkephalin, and in other ways different. They also differed from each other. Obviously, more work remained to be done on Goldstein's mysterious peptides.

While Goldstein's team kept working, so did everyone else, including Hughes and Hans Kosterlitz. Kosterlitz, then seventy-two, had been the director of the Unit for Research on Addictive Drugs at the University of Aberdeen in Scotland since 1973. Hughes worked for (and with) him. Kosterlitz was one of the great figures of his field. He'd gotten his M.D. at the University of Berlin in 1929, and his Ph.D. there in '36. He was a master at his work, and he'd won his share of awards and commendations to prove it.

In December 1975, Hughes and Kosterlitz dropped another bombshell. They had identified enkephalin. *It was part of C. H. Li's curious big protein, beta-lipotropin.* Good old seemingly-useless, sitting-on-the-shelf-for-ten-years beta-lipotropin.

More than that—there were at least two versions of enkephalin. The first kind had the amino acid methionine in the fifth position. It was referred to as "Met-enkephalin." The second one, also five amino acids long, had the amino acid leucine in the fifth position. It was called, not surprisingly, "Leu-enkephalin." It had the typical endings for such compounds, NH_2—on one end and—COOH on the other.

The sequence of Met-enkephalin was *identical to positions 61 to 65 of beta-lipotropin.* Met-enkephalin was actually beta-LPH$^{61-65}$. Like beta-MSH (which was also beta-LPH$^{41-58}$) and ACTH$^{4-10}$ (or B-LPH$^{47-53}$), Met-enkephalin seemed to be contained in a larger protein which was functioning as a precursor. It seemed likely that beta-LPH was being broken apart to make smaller compounds, like beta-MSH. Now it looked as though beta-lipotropin was also a precursor for the newly discovered endogenous peptide Met-enkephalin.

Enkephalin was a breakthrough: the first *endogenous opiate peptide* discovered. It was a *peptide* because it was a smallish molecular chain of amino acids with an amino molecular group at one end and a carboxyl at the other; *opiate* because it acted like opium compounds in the vas deferens/myenteric plexus test; and *endogenous* because it was being produced inside the body, in the brain —somewhere in the pituitary gland.

Enkephalin was also an exciting brain breakthrough because of its implications for the role of endogenous opioid chemicals in the body. A body-produced peptide that acted like morphine, a known painkiller—well, the implication was pretty obvious, and people like Hughes and Kosterlitz explicitly raised it:

Enkephalins could well be a major part of the body's pain system. The transmittal of pain information is medically known by the term "nociception." The chemical called Substance P was already thought to be a neurotransmitter of pain impulses. Could enkephalin be the body's way of *suppressing* pain?

The Endorphins

Avram Goldstein and his colleagues had two different opioid peptide substances in hand that were not enkephalins. One they had extracted from fresh cow pituitary glands, the other from a basic extract of crude ACTH taken from pig pituitaries. The stuff from the pig pituitaries would take several more years to be identified. But the chemical from the cow brain would soon be revealed as something new: an endogenous opiate that was not enkephalin.

At least three different research teams including nearly a dozen people confirmed the existence of three new opioid peptides. One of the people involved was Roger Guillemin.

Guillemin had been born in Dijon, France, in 1924. He had gotten his B.A. and B.Sc. at the University of Dijon in 1941 and 1942, and served in the French underground during the war. Afterwards, having received his M.D. at the School of Medicine in Lyons, France, in 1949, he went to Montreal, Canada. Postgraduate work followed at McGill University and the University of Montreal, and a Ph.D. in physiology and experimental medicine. While in Montreal he worked with another scientist named Andrew Schally. Both Schally and Guillemin were and are brilliant men with ambitions and egos larger than life. Such personality characteristics are neither bad nor good in themselves; what matters is how the people involved make use of them in their relationship with others and with the world. But for these two men the results were probably inevitable: colleagues at first, they ended up being competitors. The fierceness of their antagonism pushed them to greater and greater heights of scientific effort. They both desired the Nobel Prize. They both got it. Unfortunately, they had to share it with each other.

In 1952, Guillemin moved from Canada to Texas and the Baylor College of Medicine in Houston, where he remained for eighteen years. There he began his research into the mechanisms that control the chemicals secreted by the pituitary gland. It was research that involved processing more than five million sheep brains—better than fifty tons of brain tissue. It was an immense undertaking, and Schally was right with him in the race.

In 1968, Guillemin, Roger Burgus and Wylie Vale announced the finding of TRF, the first known *hypothalamic hormone*. TRF regulates the functioning of the thyroid gland by affecting the functioning of the pituitary. Days after that announcement, Schally and his team reported they had found it, too. Schally and Roger Guillemin received the Nobel Prize for this work in 1977.

In 1975, Guillemin became interested in opioid peptides.

It wasn't that surprising. Guillemin had made pituitary and hypothalamic substances his lifework. Here was something brand new. And here was a strong suggestion, from Goldstein's work, that enkephalins weren't the only new ones. In the fall of that year Guillemin and his group went to work, using the extract of two hundred and fifty thousand fragments of pig pituitary and hypothalami. Late in 1975 they found something.

Eric Simon of NYU's School of Medicine had earlier suggested that these new substances be called *endorphins*, a contraction of "endogenous morphines." Hughes and Kosterlitz had ignored that suggestion when they named their substances enkephalins. Guillemin, though, stuck to endorphins, and used the term for the first of the compounds for which he and his colleagues were able to determine an amino acid structure, or which they could characterize. They called it *alpha-endorphin*. It was a *hexadecapeptide*, sixteen amino acids long. Guillemin and his team saw at once that that alpha-endorphin was identical to the amino acid sequence in beta-lipotropin running from positions 61 to 76. And Met-enkephalin's structure was identical to the first five positions in alpha-endorphin.

More than five hundred miles to the north in San Francisco, C. H. Li and his associate David Chung had at practically the same time isolated another peptide from the extracts of those camel pituitary glands. It was identical to beta-LPH[61-91], and it possessed significant opiate-like activity. Li succeeded in making a synthetic beta-lipotropin[61-91] that was identical in activity to the stuff they got out of the camels. They submitted their results in a paper to the *Proceedings of the National Academy of Sciences*, which received it in January 1976 and published it in April. Li and Chung proposed that the newly found substance be called *beta-endorphin*.

The action wasn't confined to the west coast of the United States. Late in 1975 three British researchers had also found the last thirty-one amino acids in beta-lipotropin existing as an intact peptide in the pituitary gland. A. F. Bradbury, D. G. Smyth and

C. R. Snell worked in the Laboratory of Peptide Chemistry at London's National Institute for Medical Research. They called the peptide the "C-fragment" because it was the so-called C-terminal of beta-lipotropin, the part that ends with -COOH. The C-fragment acted like morphine. It was definitely an opioid peptide. The three submitted their results to *Nature* magazine, who got the report in February 1976 and published it in the April 29 issue that year. By then, though, the Li/Chung paper was out. The British group had come up with the same discovery as had the UCSF team, but the latter was first in the publication race. Beta-endorphin was the name, and it stuck.

Later that year, Guillemin and his team reported to the *Proceedings of the National Academy of Sciences* on the details of their discovery of alpha-endorphin. They also announced the discovery and characterization of a third peptide, which they called *gamma-endorphin*. It was almost exactly the same in structure as alpha-endorphin. It had a seventeenth amino acid—leucine—after the threonine at the end of alpha-endorphin. It was pretty obvious that C. H. Li's "useless" lipotropin was more than just an odd molecule hanging around in the brain. These relationships between the newly discovered enkephalins and endorphins on the one hand and beta-lipotropin on the other had to be more than coincidental.

In the June 1976 issue of the *Proceedings,* Guillemin, Ling and Larry Lazarus put the pieces together. They suggested that beta-lipotropin was a *prohormone,* a precursor; that the actions of various substances in the brain, such as enzymes, broke the beta-lipotropin apart into different fragments. And those fragments included the endorphin and enkephalin peptides.

In that same issue of the *Proceedings,* Avram Goldstein, C. H. Li and Brian M. Cox joined together to detail the way beta-endorphin acted like an opiate in the now standard tests. This also showed that one of the enkephalin-like substances Goldstein had found and first reported on a year ago was in fact beta-endorphin. For those who might wonder "who was first," Goldstein was first. But Guillemin was also first—the first to actually deduce the amino acid sequence of an endorphin, the first to find alpha- and gamma-endorphin, and the first to suggest a relationship between the endorphins and lipotropin. Furthermore, Li and David

Chung were first, too: the first to sequence and produce a synthetic version of beta-endorphin, and to name it. Take your pick.

At the beginning of 1976, C. H. Li had published the complete and accurate sequence for several different versions of beta-lipotropin, including the human kind. The subsequent discoveries of the endorphins presented peptides with amino acid sequences that fit right into beta-lipotropin. There were only a couple of differences in amino acids near the end, and those had to do with differences between the human and animal versions of beta-LPH and the endorphins.

Beta-endorphin was strong. While beta-lipotropin showed absolutely none of the activity of an opiate drug, beta-endorphin was 5.3 to 5.8 times as powerful as morphine. Maybe it wasn't the enkephalins that were the pain-suppressing chemicals in the brain. Perhaps it was beta-endorphin.

Beta-endorphin, at the end of 1976, was "hot." It was "sexy." It was surely a ticket to stardom in the scientific skies. Why, there might even be a Nobel Prize in it for someone.

The Year of Experiments and a Precursor

The year 1977 saw a real scramble by the people in the biochemical and brain sciences to get onto the endorphin bandwagon. People everywhere were trying to replicate and follow up some preliminary evidence in 1976 suggesting that enkephalins and endorphins not only might be the body's "natural painkillers" but also might be involved in mental illness. Other people were doing other kinds of experiments—research designed to answer more basic questions about endorphins. Questions like: Where in the brain and body are they found? How do they work (as opposed to "What might they do?")? Where do they come from? The answers to that last question, or at least the beginnings of the answer, started appearing in 1977. We're talking about precursor proteins, the source of the endorphins.

In 1975 two scientists at the University of Colorado, Richard Mains and his wife Betty Eipper, had been doing a lot of work on

ACTH. They were looking for that hormone's precursor, and they thought it might be one of several "giant ACTH" molecules. One they had begun spending a lot of time working on they called *31K-ACTH*, because it weighed thirty-one thousand daltons. It was *big*. Throughout 1975 and 1976 they continued their research, finding that ACTH was cleaved from 31K-ACTH, and also discovering evidence that beta-lipotropin, too, might be sliced from it.

In July 1977 they and Nicholas Ling of the Salk Institute announced that 31K-ACTH was indeed the precursor to ACTH, beta-lipotropin and beta-endorphin. A chemical called trypsin broke 31K-ACTH down into several fragments. One was very similar to beta-lipotropin; another fragment was similar to beta-endorphin. They could also identify in 31K-ACTH a peptide very similar to beta-lipotropin[61-69], the first nine amino acids in beta-endorphin. Also in the precursor was a sequence of amino acids identical to beta-MSH. When they examined the culture medium used to grow the cells from which they'd gotten the 31K-ACTH, they found in it approximately equimolar amounts of ACTH-related peptides and endorphin-related peptides. A similar announcement by James Roberts and Ed Herbert of the University of Oregon confirmed the discovery. Mains, Eipper and Ling had found the protein that was the precursor to ACTH, beta-lipotropin and the endorphins.

In February 1978 three researchers at the Roche Institute of Molecular Biology in Nutley, New Jersey, provided additional confirmation of the existence of the precursor. Menachem Rubinstein, Stanley Stein and Sidney Udenfriend suggested it be called *pro-opiocortin*, and that name is still often used. In 1979 another researcher, Michel Chrétien, suggested it be called *pro-opiomelanocortin* (abbreviated to POMC) to indicate that it was the precursor of beta-MSH as well as ACTH and the opioid peptides.

By 1978, then, the story of endorphins had moved rapidly forward. At the beginning of the decade few had suspected their existence. Now researchers had found not only the endorphins, but also one of the precursors of these new brain chemicals.

The Lasker Controversy

Throughout 1978 researchers continued to explore the distribution of enkephalins and endorphins in the nervous system. Others looked into possible connections the opioid peptides might have with mental illness, pain, electrical stimulation of the brain, the placebo effect and traumatic shock. No new endorphins came to light, nor was a precursor found for Leu-enkephalin. The Rubinstein/Stein/Udenfriend paper which confirmed POMC as the endorphin precursor also mentioned that the researchers had not found any of the protein with a Leu-enkephalin sequence present. So even if POMC was a Met-enkephalin precursor, it wasn't one for the other enkephalin.

Later that year, Udenfriend and his colleagues found in rat and guinea pig brains two giant opioid-containing proteins which *were not* POMC. Something else containing opioid peptide chains was floating around.

But probably the biggest news in the wonderful world of endorphins in 1978 occurred at the end of the year. It wasn't really a scandal; but one of the skeletons in science's closet began rattling.

Each year the Albert and Mary Lasker Foundation gives awards of cash and recognition to men and women in the fields of medical research and public service. They're very prestigious awards, even though the $15,000 prizes in Basic Medical Research, Applied Medical Research and Special Public Service don't come close in size to the Nobel Prize money. In fact, some scientists have said they'd rather have a Lasker than a Nobel. It's also true that many Lasker Award winners go on to win a Nobel Prize. It's been the case with nearly three dozen people at last count, including Roger Guillemin, who won a Lasker in 1975 and the Nobel two years later. Finally, while the Nobel Prize in Medicine is always limited to a maximum of three people each year, the Lasker awards have no such limit.

In November 1978 the foundation announced the winners for that year. The Basic Medical Research Award went to Solomon Snyder, John Hughes and Hans Kosterlitz, for Snyder's discovery of the opiate receptors and Hughes's and Kosterlitz's discovery. Immediately there were cries of outrage. One of the angered people had every right to be upset: Candace Pert.

Pert was now a research scientist at the National Institutes of Mental Health. But she'd been Snyder's graduate assistant during the work leading to the discovery of the opiate receptors and had collaborated with him on those experiments. In fact, her name was first on that pioneering paper and several that followed. Many followers of the field of opiate research assumed she'd been the *major* contributor, and fully expected her name to be on the list of Lasker Award recipients. Pert assumed so, too, and was "angry and upset to be excluded" from the award, as she said in a letter to Mary Lasker. "As Dr. Snyder's graduate student, I played a key role in initiating this research and following it up," Pert added. She refused an invitation to the luncheon at which the awards were presented.

Why was Pert left out in the cold? Some people, including Solomon Snyder, think it was the long-standing prejudice against graduate students. They often do all the real, dirty work in experiments directed by their mentors, but the mentors get any awards which may come out of the work. Jacob Hiller, the second author with Eric Simon of NYU on their paper reporting the opiate receptor discovery, has been quoted as saying Pert had a legitimate beef. However, her relationship with Snyder was much the same as his with Simon, he added, and Simon "was the senior investigator, and senior investigators are allowed certain privileges—like getting awards."

Nonetheless, some prickly questions remain unanswered. Why was the award limited to those particular three? Why didn't Avram Goldstein share in the award? It was his development of a method of finding the receptors which led to their being found. Why did the Lasker nominators and jurors ignore Eric Simon at NYU and Lars Terenius at Uppsala University? Their reports on the discovery of the opiate receptors and the enkephalins were nearly simultaneous with those of Snyder and Pert, and of Hughes and Kosterlitz. In fact, Terenius published his report before Hughes did, and Simon's results were submitted for publication before Terenius's.

And if the reason for Pert's exclusion was her graduate assistant relationship to Snyder, what about John Hughes? Hughes had somewhat the same relationship to Hans Kosterlitz—young scientist working with and for an older mentor—as did Pert (and

Hiller, with Eric Simon). Hughes got part of the Lasker; Pert did not. Why not?

Given the people who *did* get the 1978 Laskers, the most glaring thing about Pert's omission is not her graduate student status, but her sex. There's evidence she didn't get the award because she wasn't even *nominated* for it. The man who nominated Snyder (his department chair) has said it never occurred to him to nominate Pert. It certainly occurred to someone to nominate Hughes, but Hughes was a *male* researcher working for a senior mentor.

In a letter to *Science News* and later to *Science* magazine, the director of the Division of Research of the National Institute on Drug Abuse, Dr. William Pollin, noted that the 1977 NIDA Pacesetter Research Awards went to Snyder, Hughes and Kosterlitz—*and also* Eric Simon, Lars Terenius and Avram Goldstein for their work on opiate receptors and opioid peptides. Pert was not mentioned, he admitted, and that was later perceived as a "serious mistake" and "omission." Pollin said her graduate status was the reason at the time. Yet John Hughes was included in their awards; the only major contributor left out was a woman. In a reply, six science writers for the National Center for Atmospheric Research claimed the Pert exclusion was just one more "serious mistake" in a science-wide pattern of such exclusions.

Snyder himself has said that it would have been appropriate for Pert to be included in the Lasker awards. In a 1982 interview with *Omni* magazine, Pert says she harbors no ill feelings against Snyder, whom she's long admired and personally liked. However, one scientist at the heart of the opioid peptide field has told this author that six years afterwards Pert is still angry about the Lasker affair.

Perhaps the thing that rankles the most is the connection between the Laskers and the Nobel prizes. A large percentage of Lasker winners go on to receive the Nobel, so Snyder, Kosterlitz and Hughes can reasonably expect to get the Big One sometime soon. And the Nobel *is* limited to three per year in each science category. Where does this leave Candace Pert? Then there is the matter of who nominates people for the Laskers and the Nobels. The answer is, the same people: the department chairs and the senior researchers in the fields involved. Despite considerable changes in societal attitudes, science remains very much an "old boy" network. The people who never thought of nominating Candace Pert for a Lasker will never think of nominating her for a Nobel. There is also a strain of self-fulfilling prophesy involved, too. "She was passed over for the Lasker," some might say. "So perhaps her work isn't good enough for the Nobel."

Dr. Pert does have a strong ego; one has to if one is to be at the forefront of one's field—and she is. Strong egos are very much a privilege of famous scientists and Nobel Prize winners. Roger Guillemin is probably one of the best examples. But in other ways Pert is not exactly the stereotype of the Nobel Prize winner. Not only is she not male, she is not elderly; and she is a mother of three children.

Only time will tell if Candace Pert will receive the ultimate recognition for her co-discovery of the opiate receptors. However, it's highly likely that if she does stand before the assembled Swedish Academy and the King, it will not be in the company of Solomon Snyder, John Hughes and Hans Kosterlitz.

The " 'Big' Enkephalins"

The next endorphin breakthrough happened in 1979. A new opioid peptide, the first to be found since beta-endorphin, was announced in January. The discoverers were Japanese. Their names were Kenji Kangawa, Hisayuki Matsuo and Masao Igarashi. Kangawa and Matsuo were scientists at Miyazaki Medical College and Igarashi was at the Gunma University School of Medicine. What they found was a " 'big' Leu-enkephalin," an opioid peptide that included Leu-enkephalin in its amino acid sequence. All the other known opioid peptides could be called " 'big' Met-enkephalins," since they all included Met-enkephalin in themselves. The three researchers named their new find *alpha-neo-endorphin*—the first ("alpha") of a new ("neo") class of endorphins.

Kangawa, Matsuo and Igarashi did it the hard way, the way Guillemin and Schally had found their hypothalamic hormone-releasing factors; the way Li had found beta-lipotropin and later beta-endorphin. They processed the hypothalamus glands of pigs. Lots of them. Some thirty thousand of them. That's a lot of pigs, and a lot of pig brains cut apart, and a lot of very tiny hypothalami to be mashed and processed. It was still the only way to do it. From the extracts of thirty thousand pig hypothalami the three researchers had come up with a mere fifty micrograms (or eighteen millionths of an ounce) of alpha-neo-endorphin. But it was enough to determine that they had something different and new. They were even able to determine part of the amino acid sequence of the new peptide, though they weren't sure about the last part. It was definitely different from beta-endorphin.

It was an important breakthrough. For the first time an endogenous opioid peptide had been found that included the Leu-enkephalin sequence. Its discovery suggested the existence of a Leu-enkephalin precursor distinct from the one (POMC) for Met-enkephalin and the endorphins.

The guinea pig ileum test for opiate activity showed alpha-neo-endorphin to be 6.7 times as potent as Met-enkephalin and 5 times as potent as beta-endorphin. Alpha-neo-endorphin turned out to be the most potent of all the known endorphins.

Dynorphin, the "Dynamite" Endorphin

Alpha-neo-endorphin held its place of primacy for less than a year. Avram Goldstein was not a man to give up on a sticky problem. The problem was what he called his "type B endorphin" or "slow-reversing endorphin." It was the second of the two opioid peptides he had discovered some four years earlier, at nearly the same time that others had found the two enkephalins. Goldstein's first peptide had turned out to be beta-endorphin. The second one had remained stubbornly unidentified.

Goldstein now knew a lot about his "slow-reversing endorphin": it didn't seem to contain a methionine residue in some tests, suggesting it might contain a Leu-enkephalin sequence; its apparent molecular weight was only about half that of beta-endorphin, so it might well be a smaller molecule; its action upon the myenteric plexus of guinea pigs and rats (a test, we recall, of opiate potency) reversed only slowly when it was washed out of the tissue—thus the name "slow-reversing endorphin." Goldstein had found all that out by 1976. Since then he'd been working to get a sample pure enough for an unambiguous amino acid sequence. It took a long time.

The compound was extremely potent in opiate tests, and that meant he was working with quantities smaller than he first expected. And he also really *did* have a sticky problem. The stuff tended to be adsorbed by the glass of tubes and flasks. Adsorption means "adhesion by a gas or liquid to the surface of a solid" (*Taber's Cyclopedic Medical Dictionary, 14th edition, 1981*). In other words, it stuck to the glass and was difficult to get out. Goldstein was working with quantities measured in micrograms, and when you do that you need every particle you can get hold of.

By the middle of 1979 he had shown that the chemical was concentrated fairly strongly in the posterior lobe of the pituitary gland. And he finally had enough to begin determining the substance's amino acid sequence.

In December 1979, Goldstein and four associates announced the identity of the peptide first found in 1975. It was thirteen amino acids long, essentially Leu-enkephalin with eight additional amino acids. The peptide's potency was incredible: in the guinea pig ileum test it was *seven hundred times more potent than Leu-enkephalin.* Because of this extraordinary opiate potency, Goldstein decided to name it *dynorphin (dyn-* from the Greek *dynamis,* or "power"): "powerful endorphin."

Like alpha-neo endorphin, dynorphin was a "big Leu-enkephalin." The total amino acid sequence of that peptide wasn't yet fully known, so it wasn't yet possible to say if there was any structural relationship between the two, as there was between the endorphins, Met-enkephalin and beta-lipotropin.

The discovery of dynorphin capped an eventful 1979 for followers of endorphins, but it was by no means the end of things. Sid Udenfriend and his associates at the Roche Institute published a number of papers on their continuing work to track down the enkephalin precursor. They were finding a lot of interesting enkephalin-like peptides and larger opioid non-endorphin pep-

tides, and they were finding them in the adrenal glands of experimental animals.

The other major advance in 1979 was announced in March of
that year. A Japanese/American team determined the complete
amino acid sequence of POMC, the endorphin precursor, and
they did it in an exciting new way—genetic sequencing. Led by
Shigetada Nakanishi of the Kyoto University Faculty of Medicine,
the seven researchers spliced a piece of cattle DNA which contained the genetic code for POMC into a bacterium's plasmid.
(As we noted in the first chapter, DNA is the key to life on earth.
Usually it is found in the nucleus of a cell, but not always. A
plasmid is a ring of DNA which exists outside the cell's nucleus
and is important in moving the genetic codes out to the working
part of the cell, where they can make enzymes, amino acids and
other chemicals.) The genetically altered bacteria produced a lot
of POMC. In fact, they made enough so that the team, using a
special procedure, could finally work out the actual sequence of
nucleotide codons in DNA which governed the formation of
POMC. In other words, they cracked the POMC genetic code and
read it out to produce the amino acid sequence of that precursor.
They named the entire precursor protein they found *pre-POMC*.
It was a very important achievement, and pointed the way to new
methods of discovery in the world of endorphin research.

Enkephalin on Center Stage

Throughout 1980, Sidney Udenfriend and his colleagues at the
Roche Institute of Molecular Biology pressed their search for the
enkephalin precursor. It was now pretty obvious that neither
Met- nor Leu-enkephalin came from POMC. There were also the
two "big Leu-enkephalins" that had already been found, dynorphin and alpha-neo-endorphin, two cases where Leu-enkephalin was embedded in larger peptides. In March 1980 the
Roche team announced they had discovered still more large
opioid peptides ("enkephalin-containing peptides," or "ECPs")
which could be connected with the enkephalin precursor. They

named them *Peptide F* and *Peptide I,* and they published partial amino acid sequences for them. Peptide I had a Met- and a Leu-enkephalin inside it; Peptide F had two Met-enkephalins. The hypothesis was that they were intermediate peptides, part of the pathway from the enkephalin precursor to enkephalin. Udenfriend and friends were closing in on their quarry.

They bagged it soon after. In the June 27, 1980, issue of *Science,* the team of Randolph Lewis, Alvin Stern, Sadao Kimura, Jean Rossier, Stanley Stein and Udenfriend announced they had found what seemed to be the precursor molecule of the enkephalins: *proenkephalin.* It was a protein with a molecular weight of about fifty thousand daltons which they obtained from the adrenal glands (to be precise, from the adrenal medullas) of beef cattle. When the researchers treated their samples of the protein with two enzymes (trypsin and carboxypeptidase), the molecule broke down and produced Met- and Leu-enkephalin in a ratio of seven to one. That seemed to show proenkephalin contained seven copies of Met-enkephalin and one copy of Leu-enkephalin. The actual sequence of amino acids in proenkephalin wasn't yet known.

Udenfriend, Lewis and the others weren't the only ones in the field, though. In August two of the scientists who had discovered alpha-neo-endorphin, Kenji Kangawa and Hisayuki Matsuo, and several other colleagues reported finding an enkephalin-containing peptide they named *BAM-12P,* for "bovine adrenal medulla [its location] twelve-amino-acid-long peptide." It contained a Met-enkephalin inside it. At the end of the year they found two more large ECPs. They named them *BAM-20P* and *BAM-22P.* BAM-20P was just a shortened version of BAM-22P, and the latter peptide also contained within it the sequence for BAM-12P. BAM-12P was also part of Udenfriend's Peptide I. Udenfriend published a likely sequence for Peptide I, and there, following the Met-enkephalin sequence, was the string of amino acids that made it correspond to BAM-12P.

The discoveries continued. In 1981, Udenfriend and his associates announced finding and sequencing *Peptide B,* weighing thirty-six hundred daltons, and *Peptide E,* weighing thirty-two hundred daltons. Kangawa, Matsuo and others came up with the complete amino acid sequence for alpha-neo-endorphin, and also found another peptide floating around which they called (not surprisingly) *beta-neo-endorphin.* It turned out to be nothing more than alpha-neo-endorphin missing its last amino acid.

Near the end of 1981, Avram Goldstein and his team published what appeared to be the complete amino acid sequence for dynorphin. It had seventeen amino acids, not thirteen. But the already known first thirteen were the ones that made dynorphin as potent as it was. Still, it was an important advance.

The biggest breakthrough of 1981 came from the people in New Jersey, at the Roche Institute. It was the coming together of DNA and enkephalins.

Breaking the Enkephalin Codes

It had already been done for endorphins in 1979, when the Japanese/American research team had broken the DNA genetic code for POMC and used it to produce the complete amino acid sequence for that giant precursor molecule. What can be done once, can be done again. Udenfriend and company published a report showing a partial sequence from the messenger RNA (or mRNA) code for the enkephalin precursor, or proenkephalin. While DNA carries the primary code for an organism and everything within it, including its peptides, proteins, hormones and other chemicals, those instructions are delivered to the parts of the cell that make the stuff via messenger RNA. The mRNA code, therefore, can be just as important to break as the DNA code. Figuring out the RNA code leads right back to the original DNA code. That, in turn, leads to understanding how and why cells make the chemicals they make, and how and why they sometimes malfunction. And that has enormous implications.

The actual process by which the genetic code for endorphins was figured out is something best left for later in the book. Suffice it to say, though, that the process is incredibly time-consuming, delicate and fraught with the possibility of error. That Udenfriend and his group could come up with even a partial reading of the mRNA code for proenkephalin was a great triumph.

The triumph was soon overshadowed.

First, Ed Herbert and Michael Comb of the University of Oregon, with Roberto Crea of Genentech, Inc., in San Francisco, announced at the beginning of January 1982 that they too had determined part of the mRNA sequence that codes for enkephalin.

Then, between the end of January and February, it all broke loose. An eight-person Japanese team led by Masaharu Noda announced it had figured out the *entire* complementary DNA (or cDNA) code for *pre-proenkephalin,* the molecule that contains the precursor. The team reconstructed the entire amino acid sequence for pre-proenkephalin. The whole thing, excluding introductory sequences and follow-on sequences, was 263 amino acids long. It held within it four copies of Met-enkephalin and one copy each of Leu-enkephalin and two slightly longer versions of Met-enkephalin. The team included Shigetada Nakanishi of the Kyoto University School of Medicine—one of the seven researchers who in 1978 had found and broken the DNA code for the endorphin precursor pre-POMC.

The same issue of *Nature* that contained the Noda et al. report had one by Ueli Gubler, Sid Udenfriend and three other teammates. They, too, had done what the Japanese had done. But the editors of *Nature* had received the Japanese report first, so they gave it primacy of place.

That wasn't the end of it, though. A month later, in the same magazine, Herbert and Comb of the University of Oregon, along with colleagues from Genentech and the National Institutes of Health, reported *their* uncoding of the mRNA for the enkephalin precursor. They showed it to be 267 amino acids long, not 263, and they noted where Peptide B, Peptide E and Peptide F were in the DNA/amino acid sequence. Herbert and company had made the breakthrough at the same time as the other two teams had; in fact, they may even have been first—the time sequence is difficult to reconstruct. What angered Herbert was that the *Nature* editors had apparently promised him his paper would be published along with the other two, in the same issue. It wasn't, and Herbert and his people looked like johnny-come-latelies, which they certainly weren't.

Discovery of Pre-Prodynorphin

The discovery and announcement of pre-proenkephalin was just the first punch of a double-whammy delivered by the Japanese researchers. On July 15, 1982, they announced their discovery and sequencing of the dynorphin/alpha-neo-endorphin precursor. The discovery team was essentially the same as the one which found pre-proenkephalin. Again it included Shigetada Nakanishi, who was in on the discovery and sequencing of all three of the known opioid peptide precursors. They referred to the en-kephalin precursor as *pre-proenkephalin A,* and to the dynorphin/ alpha-neo-endorphin precursor as *pre-proenkephalin B.* However, "pre-proenkephalin B" implies that the protein is a second en-kephalin precursor, something not known to be true. Brian Cox of the Uniformed Services University of the Health Sciences in Bethesda, Maryland, and one of Goldstein's collaborators, has suggested "pre-prodynorphin" as a better name for the mole-cule. The pre-prodynorphin genetic code contains 2,333 nucleo-tides. Pre-prodynorphin itself has at least 257 amino acids. So it's about the same size as POMC and pre-proenkephalin.

Still More Endorphins

As 1982 came to an end, Goldstein and several associates at the Addiction Research Foundation and Stanford University an-nounced the discovery of two new opioid peptides, "big" dy-norphins. The new molecules were isolated from the pituitary glands of pigs, those now venerable and unsung contributors to the endorphin revolution. The first was twenty-four amino acids long and included the complete dynorphin-17 sequence at its beginning. Following it were seven more amino acids: lysine, arginine and then a Leu-enkephalin sequence.

The second "big" dynorphin was thirty-two amino acids long. It included all of dynorphin-24 plus a little bit more. The last thirteen amino acids (dynorphin[20-32]) were separated from the first seventeen (dynorphin[1-17]) by the amino acid duo of lysine and arginine, which Goldstein and others consider a cleaving site. So Goldstein decided dynorphin[20-32] could legitimately be considered a new and separate dynorphin. He named that sequence *dynorphin-B.*

The year ended with another publication from the Roche Institute people. Udenfriend and his associates announced in November the discovery of another new endorphin they called *rimorphin.* It was thirteen amino acids long and was present in parts of the posterior pituitary glands of cattle. They found it associated with both dynorphin and alpha-neo-endorphin, and they claimed rimorphin has a structure unlike the other two. It turned out, though, that rimorphin wasn't new after all: it was actually dynorphin B. It wasn't a total loss for the Roche group, because they were the first to find it in the brain.

By 1983, twelve years after Avram Goldstein suggested a way to find opiate receptors in the brain, ten years after those receptors were found, and a mere eight years after the announcement of the discovery of the first known endogenous opioid peptide, science knew of at least three different "classes" of endorphins:

• the *enkephalins,* Met- and Leu-;
• the *endorphins* proper: alpha-, gamma- and beta-;
• the *dynorphins,* -13, -17 (or -A), -24, -32, -8, -B and other fragments, and *alpha-neo-endorphin.*

There was also a scattering of large enkephalin-containing opioid peptides that were probably intermediate molecules in the breakdown of the enkephalin precursor.

And there were the precursors:

• *pro-opiomelanocortin,* or POMC, the endorphin precursor;
• *pre-proenkephalin,* the enkephalin precursor;
• *pre-prodynorphin,* the precursor to the dynorphins and the -neo-endorphins.

4

Origins and Destinations

The opioid peptides, the endorphins, enkephalins and dynorphins, begin their existence as parts of larger proteins called precursors. They end their existence fitting into tiny "keyholes" in cell membranes, places called receptors. Let's pause a bit here to look in a little more detail at the origins and destinations of the endorphins.

Process, and a Problem

For many years neurochemists have known that some of the chemicals present in the body, especially hormones like insulin, epinephrine, and dopamine, themselves were originally parts of larger molecules called prohormones or precursors. The smaller hormones and peptides were cleaved or "sliced" out of these larger proteins by the action of other chemicals called enzymes, which are much like catalysts: they cause changes in another substance without being changed themselves. A substance that's an enzyme is usually identified by the suffix *-ase*. Lipases are enzymes that split fats; proteinases break down proteins; peptidases do the same to peptides. Two of the best-known enzymes, rennin and trypsin, were named before the -ase rule was adopted.

It seemed pretty reasonable to assume that the newly discovered endogenous opioid peptides were also the products of larger precursor proteins, and were cleaved out by enzymes or enzyme-like chemicals. A number of scientists including Roger Guillemin and C. H. Li had already suggested that beta-lipotropin was a precursor of the endorphins and Met-enkephalin. Certainly the amino acid sequences for these endorphins were completely present inside lipotropin.

There was, however, a problem with Met-enkephalin. The last two amino acids in beta-lipotropin just before the beginning of the endorphin sequence were lysine and arginine. Abundant evidence existed that the chemical bond between these two was weak and easily broken. So it was pretty likely that the beta-endorphin molecule (with its enclosed alpha- and gamma- sequences) was cleaved off of beta-lipotropin. However, the amino acids following the (position 5) methionine of the Met-enkephalin sequence at the beginning of the endorphin sequence were thrionine and serine. They had a much stronger chemical bond, one not easily broken. That made it unlikely that Met-enkephalin was cleaved from beta-lipotropin.

And what about beta-lipotropin itself? It was ninety-one amino acids long, a reasonably large-sized protein. But did it have a precursor, too? Past experience suggested it would. Past experience proved correct.

The Endorphin Precursor

Though enkephalins were the first-discovered endogenous peptides, the first endogenous peptide precursor to be identified and sequenced was the one for beta-endorphin. That was beta-lipotropin, found in 1964 by Choh Hao Li and eleven years later recognized as beta-endorphin's precursor almost simultaneously with that peptide's discovery. It soon became apparent, though, that beta-lipotropin wasn't the final answer. Researchers discovered that the pituitary gland released beta-endorphin and ACTH simultaneously. That strongly hinted at a common origin for the two chemicals. Richard Mains and Betty Eipper of the University of Colorado found several large proteins that seemed to contain either ACTH or beta-endorphin/beta-lipotropin. In 1977 they were finally able to announce that one of those proteins, with a molecular weight of about thirty-one thousand daltons (the 31K precursor), seemed to contain both ACTH and beta-endorphin. Early in 1978, Menachem Rubinstein, Stanley Stein and Sid Udenfriend specifically identified amino acid sequences in the 31K protein which corresponded to known sequences of opioid peptides, or parts of opioid peptides. They suggested it be called *pro-opiocortin*, since it contained both ACTH and beta-endorphin. Later the name was changed to *pro-opiomelanocortin*, recognizing the protein's function as the precursor of MSH. Usually it's just called POMC; it's shorter and easier to say.

At least two research teams worked at determining the complete amino acid sequence of POMC by using a cDNA clone and "reading out" the precursor's genetic code. They were Shigetada Nakanishi and his associates at the Kyoto University Faculty of Medicine, and James Roberts at UCSF and Ed Herbert at the University of Oregon, and their associates. This approach was a major breakthrough, and signaled the way the enkephalin precursor would later be characterized. Both teams worked through 1978, trying to crack the DNA code which signaled the neurons in the pituitary gland to make POMC. On January 29, 1979, the Roberts/Herbert team submitted a paper to the *Proceedings of the National Academy of Sciences*, reporting the successful partial sequencing of POMC. On the same day, the Nakanishi team's report was received by *Nature* magazine. The Japanese, it turned out, had gone the distance, and had successfully sequenced the entire POMC protein. They were thus able to pinpoint the exact locations of ACTH and beta-lipotropin in the precursor, and accurately predict the locations of the remaining amino acids.

There are 1,091 nucleotides making up the cDNA that codes for pre-POMC. Each amino acid, recall, is represented by one or more combinations of three nucleotides called codons. Pre-POMC contains 265 amino acids. The remaining 296 nucleotides are in sequences preceding and following the pre-POMC precursor itself. The first 131 amino acids in pre-POMC contain a 26-

amino-acid "signal sequence" at the beginning, followed by a 105-amino-acid peptide called the "pro-sequence." Within the pro-sequence there seems to be a sequence corresponding to the hormone gamma-MSH. The second half of pre-POMC, the last 134 amino acids (403 nucleotides), include the complete sequences for ACTH, CLIP (corticotropin-like intermediate [lobe] protein), alpha-MSH, beta-lipotropin, beta-MSH and beta-endorphin. Within beta-endorphin, of course, are the sequences for alpha- and gamma-endorphin. Here, too, is a Met-enkephalin sequence, though by now it was apparent to most researchers that Met-enkephalin didn't come from the endorphin precursor.

Guy Boileau, Nabil Seidah and Michel Chrétien determined the breakdown sequences that lead from pre-POMC to beta-endorphin. Essentially, pre-POMC first breaks down into two fragments. One weighs about twenty-five to twenty-seven thousand daltons and is essentially the pre-sequence fragment and ACTH together. The other is beta-lipotropin. Then the 25–27K fragment is cleaved into the pre-sequence fragment and ACTH. ACTH may then be broken down to alpha-MSH and CLIP. Meanwhile, beta-lipotropin will eventually be fragmented to gamma-lipotropin (the first thirty-nine amino acids in beta-lipotropin) and beta-endorphin. Gamma-lipotropin may eventually break down still further, to beta-MSH.

The separations happen at specific points in the pre-POMC compound called "proteolytic cleavage sites." "Proteolytic" is a word applied to proteins susceptible to separation via chemical actions involving water. It's a common process in many proteins. These sites in the protein or peptide are specific pairs of amino acids that Avram Goldstein calls "putative processing sites." They are lysine-arginine, arginine-lysine, lysine-lysine, and arginine-arginine. Not all instances of these pairs turn out to be cleaving regions in proteins—but a lot of them do.

The Enkephalin Precursor

The precursor protein for Met-enkephalin was initially thought to be beta-lipotropin. The Met-enkephalin sequence is embedded within it, and is also the first five amino acids of the three endorphins, which are definitely cleaved out of beta-lipotropin. However, it soon became evident that Met-enkephalin was not likely to be derived from beta-lipotropin. For one thing, the enkephalins have a distribution in the CNS which is quite different from that of beta-endorphin, something which would be unlikely if the two had the same precursor. Then there was the matter of how easy or difficult it would be for Met-enkephalin to be broken off of the beta-endorphin molecule. It turned out to be chemically rather unlikely. The two amino acids following the Met-enkephalin sequence, threonine and serine, are held together with a strong chemical bond. There is no known process by which that bond is easily broken in normal day-to-day biochemical operations. And, of course, there was Leu-enkephalin, which is not part of the beta-lipotropin/beta-endorphin sequence at all. Where did *it* come from?

The enkephalins, it turns out, come from a rather large protein called *pre-proenkephalin*. Its discovery was announced in January 1982 by Ed Herbert, Michael Comb and Roberto Crea, and by a Japanese team led by Masaharu Noda and including the pre-POMC co-discoverer Shigetada Nakanishi. They used genetic engineering techniques to clone the DNA for the precursor and to figure out its composition and structure. Its molecular weight is about thirty-one thousand, similar to that of the endorphin precursor molecule. Pre-proenkephalin has 267 amino acids in it. The first twenty-four are the signal peptide. Following that, from positions 25 to 97, is a 73-amino-acid peptide with no name. It includes six cysteines, an amino acid which contains sulfur. Chemical bonds called disulfide bridges allow this part of the molecule to fold over, so that the precursor can be processed more efficiently by the appropriate cleaving molecules. Pre-proenkephalin includes one copy of Leu-enkephalin, four copies of Met-enkephalin, Met-enkephalin-Arg[6]-Gly[7]-Leu[8], and Met-enkephalin-Arg[6]-Phe[7]. All seven of these enkephalins are flanked on both ends by the amino acid processing signals.

Ed Herbert and the University of Oregon team, one of the

discoverers of the pre-proenkephalin sequence, examined the huge molecule very carefully with an eye to finding sequences for other "enkephalin-containing" peptides. Nowhere in pre-proenkephalin did they find amino acid sequences for dynorphin, alpha-neo-endorphin or beta-endorphin. Of course, researchers knew beta-endorphin came from pre-POMC, but it was still worthwhile taking a look at pre-proenkephalin, too. Dynorphin and alpha-neo-endorphin were more realistic expectations. They have Leu-enkephalin sequences within them, and were already known to be absent from pre-POMC. That they didn't turn up in pre-proenkephalin, either, strengthened the belief of some scientists that they were indeed a third and separate "genus" of endogenous opiates, with their own precursor molecule and neuronal pathways.

Herbert and company did find other ECPs inside pre-proenkephalin. These included the large "alphabetic" peptides found by the Udenfriend team at the Roche Institute for Molecular Biology, Peptides B, E, F and I; and the "BAM" peptides found by Kenji "alpha-neo-endorphin" Kangawa and the rest of his team of Japanese researchers—Bam 12P, -20P and -22P. Peptide F, with Met-enkephalins at the beginning and end, corresponds to positions 107 to 140 in the enkephalin precursor. Peptide B, containing a Met-enkephalin, is positions 238 to 267 in pre-proenkephalin. Peptide I, thirty-nine amino acids long, contains a Met- and a Leu-enkephalin. Peptide I is the same as pre-proenkephalin[196-234]. Peptide E, with a Met-enkephalin at the beginning and a Leu-enkephalin at the end, is a shortened version of Peptide I. Its sequence runs from positions 210 to 234 in the precursor. The three BAM peptides are also shortened versions of Peptide I. In fact, they are shortened versions of Peptide E. BAM-12P is positions 210 to 221; BAM-20P, positions 210 to 229; BAM-22P, positions 210 to 231.

Daniel Kilpatrick, Sid Udenfriend and the rest of the Roche team had long believed that the large enkephalin-containing peptides they were finding in the adrenal medulla were intermediate products in the "biosynthetic pathway" from an enkephalin precursor to enkephalin. Mizuno and Kangawa assumed the same thing. They were all correct. The different intermediate peptides are separated from each other within pre-proenkephalin by the paired amino acids Lys-Lys, Lys-Arg, Arg-Lys, or Arg-Arg, the "cleavage signals" often found within proteins and peptides.

The Dynorphin Precursor

The most recent opioid precursor to be found is the one for dynorphin and alpha-neo-endorphin. The same team that found the enkephalin precursor found this one, and once again Shigetada Nakanishi was there. Again, they successfully used genetic engineering techniques, with a "library" of DNA clones to determine the nature and sequence of the precursor. The discoverers called the precursor *pre-proenkephalin B*, but because that's a bit misleading (we don't know for sure that it is a precursor to enkephalins), it's probably better to refer to it as *pre-prodynorphin*.

Pre-prodynorphin contains 257 amino acids, and its DNA code has 2,333 nucleotides. It is similar in structure to the other two opioid precursors; the size is similar; it has an introductory signal sequence of about the same size; it contains six so-called "disulphide bonds," which cause the molecule to fold up in such a way that it can be easily sliced up by enzymatic action at the appropriate cleaving points; and it has within itself a number of amino acid sequences which duplicate each other. All these similarities suggest the three precursors have a common molecular ancestor. Long ago, perhaps a billion years or more in the past, the original "opioid precursor molecule" existed inside some one-celled creature, producing something analogous to opioid peptides for who knows what purpose.

The pre-prodynorphin precursor also has something the other two do not: a very long "tail" of still undeciphered nucleotides. As of this writing it had not been figured out, and no one knows whether there are other, still undiscovered dynorphins lurking within it.

Pre-prodynorphin, however, does contain the sequences for all the known dynorphin peptides. It also has the sequence for alpha- (and beta-)neo-endorphin. Thus the suspicions of many researchers, including Avram Goldstein, proved out: the two peptides are indeed related to each other.

Biosynthesis

The journey from precursor protein to final opioid peptide probably goes through several separate steps.

• First, the genetic code for the precursor gets passed from DNA to messenger RNA, or mRNA, which synthesizes the amino acid groups in the cytoplasm of the cell. Then transfer RNA, or tRNA, carries the amino acid groups to another part of the cell called ribosomes. These extremely tiny structures in the cell are protein factories. Here is where the precursor protein is made.

• Now the ribosome begins manufacturing the protein using the amino acids created by the mRNA and carried to it by the tRNA. After about sixty or so amino acids have been joined together, the signal peptide has been fully created and has emerged from the part of the ribosome that's making the protein.

• The signal peptide end now helps to form a junction between the sixty-unit long chain with its attached ribosome and the *rough-surfaced endoplasmic reticulum,* or RER. The RER is part of an intricate network of microcanals running through the cell's nucleus and cytoplasm. Once the peptide chain is connected the protein synthesis process continues until the entire precursor is formed from the amino acids. The signal peptide gets cut off.

• The entire precursor protein now is passed on from the RER to a place in the cell called the Golgi complex. It sounds like the title of some secret Russian rocket launching site. What it is, is a set of curved, flattened sacs near the nucleus of almost all cells. The Golgi complex is a warehouse; it stores proteins or other compounds that the cell will later secrete.

• From the Golgi complex the precursor is transported to condensing vacuoles, tiny spaces in the cell where the up-to-now dilute protein solution gets concentrated. While it's being moved from the Golgi complex, the precursor will be broken down into its various active peptides by chemicals attacking it at its different amino acid processing sites.

· Finally, the conglomeration of precursor, intermediate peptides and end-product arrives at its final destination. This may be the vesicles at the end of neuronal axons if the final product is a neurotransmitter. Or it may be secretion granules, from which secretory proteins such as hormones are released.

And when it gets to the synaptic vesicle, the neurotransmitter —now fully broken out of its precursor—will wait. Wait for the electrical wave sweeping down the length of the neuron. Wait for the vesicle to pop. And it does, and the chemical is released into the gap. Swiftly it crosses the synapse, and finds on the other side the membrane of another neuron. Are there receptor sites for it? There are.

The Opioid Receptor Sites

As we saw in Chapter 1, the opioid peptides plug into places on the neurons called receptor sites in much the same way a key fits into a lock. But what's the precise method by which chemicals like beta-endorphin and heroin turn on the opiate receptor? Why do the opiate receptor sites work for both exogenous and endogenous opiates? The answer lies first of all in the structure, the "architecture" if you will, of the chemicals.

Scientists have determined the physical structure of opiate drugs by means of X-ray diffraction, in effect by taking X-ray pictures of the crystallized form of the drug and then deducing the positions of the atoms in the molecule by the way those atoms deflected the X-rays. The natural, semisynthetic and synthetic versions of the opiates—morphine, heroin, methadone, levorphanol and others—all have very similar structures. Their structures are in fact a large part of the reason for their opiate activity. The relative placement of the atoms in the molecules makes it possible for parts of the molecules to physically and chemically fit into the neurons' opiate receptor sites.

So it came as no surprise when the newly discovered "natural opiates" called enkephalins, though larger than the opiate drugs like morphine or methadone, turned out to have structures similar in part to the more well-known opiate drugs. They had to. One important part of the enkephalin structure turned out to be the placement of the amino acid named tyrosine.

Tyrosine (or "Tyr," as scientists abbreviate it) is in a terminal rather than internal position in the enkephalins. It's at one of the two ends: to be precise, the amino or *N-terminal,* where two atoms of hydrogen and one of nitrogen in the form "NH_2—" attach. Because tyrosine is sitting there rather than inside the molecule, its nitrogen atom is not completely involved in chemical bonds. In the parlance of chemistry, it is a *basic nitrogen;* it is capable of forming chemical bonds with hydrogen ions (protons; positively charged subatomic particles). To get a bit more chemical, the nitrogen in tyrosine is an *anion.* It carries a negative charge, which is why it's attracted to positively charged hydrogen ions. The chemical bond it can form is called an *anionic bond.*

These are two characteristics held in common by the opioid peptides and the opiate alkaloid drugs: the physical structure with tyrosine at the N-terminal; and the nature of that terminal which makes it basic and able to form anionic bonds. As to why both exogenous and endogenous opiates are able to act in similar fashion, an explanation has been suggested by Avram Goldstein.

On the basis of work done by himself and others, Goldstein postulates a "message-address" concept of the way opiate drugs and opioid peptides work with the opiate receptors. The message of an opioid peptide is the sequence of amino acids which actually has opioid activity. The address is the part of the peptide that specifies which particular opioid receptor will be occupied by the peptide.

In the case of all the endorphin peptides, the message is the first four amino acids in the sequence. And the key to that message, Goldstein says, is tyrosine, hanging out there at the beginning with its basic nitrogen—for the opiate receptors on the membrane of the neuron all have a "tetrapeptide pocket," says Goldstein, a part that has an anionic site into which the basic nitrogen of the N-terminal tyrosine can fit (and also a hydrogen bond acceptor for another part of the tyrosine molecule). Here the message of the first four amino acids can fit. Here, too, can fit the structurally similar part of morphine, heroin, methadone, levorphanol, and the other exogenous opiate drugs. The message is "opiate activity." The message gets through.

The rest of the peptide, the part that follows the first four amino acids, is the "address." This is what determines *which type* of opiate receptor the peptide will plug into.

What do receptors actually look like? Well, we don't have a picture of one. Yet. But some people are working at it. A little over a year ago three scientists at the Hormone Research Lab in San Francisco (R. Glenn Hammonds, Pierre Nicolas and C. H. Li) took a step toward physically characterizing a structure in rat brain membranes that acts as a beta-endorphin receptor. Using techniques much too complicated to describe here, the three determined that the receptor/beta-endorphin complex has a shape equivalent to an elliptical spheroid—something like an egg, but not quite. It has a total molecular weight of about six hundred ninety thousand daltons. And that is *huge*. Pre-POMC is only about one four-hundredth the size of the beta-endorphin receptor.

Types of Receptors

Before the endorphins and their receptors were ever discovered, researchers had already known that other neuroregulatory chemical systems in the CNS used two or more types of receptors. That fact suggested that there would be more than one opiate receptor. Then, too, there is the undeniable fact that morphine-like drugs cause a whole constellation of effects in the creatures that receive them. Not only do they induce analgesia; they also can depress breathing and induce the state we call addiction, or drug dependence. Being deprived of them results in withdrawal symptoms. One class of synthetic opiate drugs called benzomorphs can also cause a combination of sedation, psychosis, and a state akin to drunkenness. The symptoms of the psychosis include depersonalization, dysphoria (which is the exact opposite of euphoria), suspiciousness and hallucinations.

All these effects caused by the same chemical! It is just very difficult for biochemists and molecular pharmacologists to believe that all those effects are caused by the interaction of the chemical with just one receptor. It is more likely that several receptors are involved.

In 1976 a researcher named W. R. Martin and his colleagues postulated the existence of at least three different opiate receptor populations in the central nervous system of dogs. They called them (1) *mu receptors,* with which morphine-like drugs preferentially interacted; (2) *kappa receptors,* with which some of the benzomorph drugs interacted, including one called ketocyclazocine; and (3) *sigma receptors,* which were the receptors for a drug named SKF-10,047. Martin said that the physical effects associated with the mu receptor included the slowing down of heart action (in medical terminology called *bradycardia),* hypothermia, analgesia and indifference. Effects associated with the kappa receptor, he said, included constriction of the pupils and sedation. Associated with the sigma receptor was *tachycardia* (a rapid speedup in heart rate), the abnormal dilation of the pupil and, in dogs at least, canine delirium. Later Hans Kosterlitz and his co-workers provided evidence for a fourth opiate receptor, which they called the *delta receptor.* This was the site on neurons, they said, at which the enkephalin peptides preferentially interact.

In 1981, Solomon Snyder suggested that Met-enkephalin links up specifically with the mu receptor, and Leu-enkephalin with the delta receptor. A number of experiments indicate that beta-endorphin is perfectly happy to plug into either of those two, and does. So the mu receptor would be the one at which morphine-like drugs and also Met-enkephalin would preferentially interact; the delta receptor would be the one with which Leu-enkephalin would preferentially interact; and both would be receptors with which beta-endorphin would interact.

Now there is evidence suggesting that the mu receptor is actually two: mu_1 and mu_2. According to work done by Gavril Pasternak at the Sloan-Kettering Cancer Center and Cornell University Medical Center, the mu_1 receptor is a "high-affinity" receptor, while the mu_2 receptor and the delta receptor are "low-affinity" receptors. Given a choice, in other words, both the opiates like heroin and Met-enkephalin/beta-endorphin have a high affinity for binding with mu_1. Pasternak has also produced some evidence that the analgesic effects of morphine, the endorphins and the enkephalins are mediated through the high-affinity receptor. The depressed respiration effect of morphine, though, seems to be mediated through that chemical's interaction with the low-affinity mu_2 receptor and with the delta receptor.

While some people have wondered if the kappa and sigma receptors actually exist, there's a lot of evidence to suggest they do. In fact, Avram Goldstein and his associates, particularly Charles Chavkin, have pretty much proved that the kappa receptor is not only the receptor for some benzomorph drugs, but is in fact the natural receptor for dynorphin. Martin's experiments with the chemical SKF-10,047 are evidence of the existence of the sigma receptor. R. Suzanne and Stephen Zukin of the Albert Einstein School of Medicine have found compelling evidence of the existence of sigma opiate receptors in the brain. Several other researchers have done experiments that seem to indicate that PCP, sometimes called "angel dust," wreaks its mental havoc by interacting with an opiate receptor in the brain that is identical with the ones identified as sigma receptors.

Recent experiments have shown the endorphin/opiate receptor scene to be still more complex. Some man-made versions of the enkephalins, called enkephalin analogues, interact with other than their "natural" receptors. Most interesting is a version of Met-enkephalin called FK 33-824, which like beta-endorphin seems to fit equally well with both mu and delta receptors.

cAMPing Out at the Synapse

So far we've looked at the major mechanism for the excitation or inhibition of the neuronal membrane. However, there's another process going on inside the neuron which modifies the membrane's excitability and thus its ability to send electrical signals. It involves a chemical "ménage à trois."

ATP is the abbreviation for *adenosine triphosphate,* an extremely important chemical in all cells. When it's split apart a great deal of energy gets released to power the cell. An enzyme which works a particular change upon ATP is called adenosine $3^1,5^1$-cyclic monophosphate, or *cAMP synthetase*. It converts ATP into another chemical called *cAMP*. However, for cAMP synthetase to do this to ATP, the enzyme has to be plugged into "the bottom" of a receptor site—*and a neurotransmitter has to be plugged into the other end*. If either of the two compounds is not hooked into the receptor site, the enzyme cannot convert ATP into cAMP. But when that three-way interaction is taking place, the enzyme converts ATP into cAMP. Then cAMP activates a protein in the neuron called *kinase*. The kinase makes the membrane more excitable. That in turn makes the whole neuron less inhibited, more easily "turned on" by neurotransmitters fitting into the receptor sites.

Inhibition and Opiate Receptors

One of the more important discoveries in recent years has been how endorphins and enkephalins operate through their receptors to disinhibit some interneuron networks. In particular, George Siggins, formerly with the Salk Institute in San Diego and now at the Research Institute of Scripps Clinic in La Jolla, has done a lot of work to explain how this works. In nearly every area in which it was present, the enkephalin pentapeptide acted as if it were an inhibitory neurotransmitter. The one puzzling exception was in an area of the brain called the *hippocampus*. The hippocampus is buried deep in the brain in the part called the limbic system. Its activity has been linked to emotions, memory and the recognition of familiar objects. Part of the hippocampus is made of the so-called *pyramidal* cells (their structure, with all their branching axons, looks a little like a pyramid). These pyramidal cells, rather than being inhibited by the application of morphine-like drugs or enkephalins, were actually excited by them. Siggins (and others) showed that the process in this case was a two-step one. The enkephalins and/or opiate drugs *were* inhibiting neurons, all right. But not the pyramidal cells. Rather, they were inhibiting the action of nerve cells called interneurons which *were themselves* inhibiting the action of the pyramidal cells. The net result was to allow the pyramidal cells to fire off faster, to become excited.

Siggins showed that the distribution of opiate receptors is quite subtle in its effect on different parts of the brain. The pyramidal cells have receptors which accept the inhibitory neuro-transmitters being emitted by their associated inhibitory inter-neurons. They do not, though, seem to have opiate receptors. So the enkephalins and other opioid peptides do not inhibit their action. The inhibition is accomplished by another neurotransmit-ter, presumably GABA. The interneurons using that inhibitory neurotransmitter, however, *do* have opiate receptors, so that *they* can be slowed down by enkephalin action. Result: chemicals that inhibit neuron firing in other parts of the brain (i.e., enkephalins and endorphins) act to excite certain neurons in the hippocam-pus, a brain center for emotion and memory.

Why the brain took this particular evolutionary path, to use opiate receptors in this "double-negative" manner in part of the limbic system, is still a bit of a mystery.

How Many, and Where?

Is there some kind of exclusivity among neurons and opiate re-ceptors? Sort of a "one neuron–one receptor" arrangement? This, in fact, had been the standard operating theory for neurons and their neuromodulatory receptor sites—that each neuron car-ries only one kind of receptor: this one, for example, will have nothing but dopamine receptors; that one, just GABA receptors; the one over there, nothing but delta receptors; and this one, right here, mu_1 receptors. New research, however, has shown that some neurons in some parts of the brain carry multiple opiate receptors. Two scientists at the Max Planck Institute of Psychiatry in Munich, J. T. Williams and W. Zieglgansberger, found this to be true of neurons in the frontal cortex of rats. When they desensitized the neurons to Met-enkephalin and the synthetic version of Leu-enkephalin called DADLE, the neurons became subsensitive to morphine. However, when they did the opposite—desensitized the neurons to morphine—the cells did *not* become subsensitive or desensitized to the enkephalins. Rather, they remained sensitive to the inhibitory action of the two opioid peptides. That suggests the presence of two and possibly more types of opiate receptors on the same cell.

If this is true, it makes the interaction of neurons and the possibilities for information processing and transfer in the brain just that much more subtle. It now seems that the action of the neuron can be modified not by just one neurochemical or by an interneuron network, but by two or more chemicals at once.

Opiate receptors are found in many places in the "older" parts of the brain: in the limbic system, the hippocampus and the amygdala; in the cerebellum and medulla and in parts of the brainstem. However, the cerebral cortex also has concentrations of these receptors. A report published just a year ago by Steven Wise and Miles Herkenham of the National Institute of Mental Health pinpointed some of those places in the brains of rhesus monkeys. Parts of the cerebral cortex rich in these receptors include somatic sensory areas (somatic nerves in the body report sensory data to the brain about the skin, muscles and other tissues); and areas involved in sight and hearing. The technique which Wise and Herkenham used, called *autoradiographic visualization,* sharply outlined some of the boundaries or transitions between adjacent parts of the cerebral cortex. (Autoradiographic visualization involves thin slide-mounted slices of rhesus monkey brains, radioactively tagged naloxone and photographic film.) The variation in distribution of opiate receptors suggests to the two researchers that these receptors play an important role in the function of the cerebral cortex. And it illustrates how much more we have to learn about the functions of opiate receptors in the brain, even though it's been a full ten years since they were first discovered.

5

The Endogenous Opioid Peptides

Dozens of distinct chemicals exist in the body and brain which can be classified as "endogenous opioid peptides"—peptides produced within the body which have opiate activity of some kind or another. Borrowing (with neither permission nor authorization!) the vocabulary of taxonomic classification of living creatures, we can talk of the "family" of endogenous opioid peptides (which are part of the "class" of "neuroregulators"). Within the "family" are the different "genera"—the endorphins, the enkephalins and the dynorphins. Each "genus" of peptides comes in several natural "species." So we can talk about Leu-enkephalin and Met-enkephalin; beta-endorphin (alpha- and gamma- are incomplete fragments); and dynorphin-17 (or -A), -24, -32, -B and neo-endorphin. This scheme takes into account the precursor origins of the different opioid peptides. The enkephalins, beta-endorphin and the dynorphins each originate in a separate precursor. The only exception might be Leu-enkephalin, which could also be cleaved from pre-prodynorphin. The early "big Leu-/Met-enkephalin" suggestion of the Japanese discoverers of neo-endorphin turns out to be misleading at best.

In this chapter we'll take a close look at three genera of endogenous opioid peptides. We'll quickly recap their discovery; examine their chemical makeup and physical structure; and see where they are found in the brain and other parts of the body. We begin with the first-discovered of the opioid peptides: the enkephalins.

The Enkephalins

Discovery. Although the enkephalins, endorphins and dynorphin were all actually discovered nearly simultaneously, the enkephalins were the first to be identified by name. John Hughes of the University of Aberdeen in Scotland is generally acknowledged as the author of the first published account of enkephalin's discovery in the May 2, 1975, issue of *Brain Research*. Later that month, at the annual meeting of the International Narcotic Research Club, several more scientists announced their discovery of enkephalin. They included Lars Terenius and Agneta Wahlstrom of the University of Uppsala in Sweden, and Solomon Snyder, Gavril Pasternak and Robert Goodman of Johns Hopkins University in the United States. Hughes also reported on some additional work he and his team had been doing on the newly discovered chemical.

In December 1975, Hughes, Hans Kosterlitz and four colleagues reported they had identified enkephalin as actually being two slightly different *pentapeptides* (peptides five amino acids in length). Each had an amino N-terminal and a carboxyl or C-terminal—that is, the atoms NH_2— at one end and —$COOH$ at the other. In between were the amino acids. The first enkephalin they called *Leucine-enkephalin,* or Leu-enkephalin. The second they named *Methionine-enkephalin,* or Met-enkephalin. Both contained the amino acid tyrosine, followed by two glycines and then a phenylalanine. Leu-enkephalin ended with the amino acid leucine. Met-enkephalin ended with methionine.

Hughes and his colleagues noted that Met-enkephalin was identical to the amino acids in positions 61 to 65 in beta-lipotropin, the protein discovered in 1964 by C. H. Li and found by the end of 1975 in the pituitary glands of pigs, sheep and humans. They also pointedly referred to some of the structural relationships among the beta-lipotropin, ACTH and beta-MSH molecules. And they said it was "tempting to speculate" that some relationship might exist between beta-lipotropin and the opiate molecules already found by Goldstein but not yet named. It was a temptation too strong to resist, too. Hughes and company went right ahead and speculated. Perhaps, they wondered, beta-lipotropin was a common precursor to all those chemicals, and to Met-enkephalin as well.

As it later turned out, they were wrong about Met-enkephalin.

Composition and structure. What exactly do the enkephalins look like? One "picture" of the enkephalins uses a series of amino acid abbreviations hooked together with hyphens.

Leu-enkephalin

NH_2-Tyr-Gly-Gly-Phe-Leu-COOH

Met-enkephalin

NH_2-Tyr-Gly-Gly-Phe-Met-COOH

As we mentioned in Chapter 1, scientists often use a kind of "shorthand" to describe peptides and proteins. This shorthand uses abbreviations for the names of the amino acids and strings them together with hyphens to show their position relative to each other. In the shorthand description of Leu-enkephalin above, tyrosine (Tyr) is in position 1 in the molecule, the first position following the amino terminal. Glycines occupy positions 2 and 3, the phenylalanine is in position 4, and the leucine in position 5, followed by the carboxyl terminal. If we altered the peptide by substituting a different amino acid for one of the standard ones, we'd write the description out by first giving the new amino acid's abbreviation; then its position number in superscript following it; and then the name of the peptide itself. Leu-enkephalin with an alanine in position 2 would be called [Ala²]-Leu-enkephalin, for example. Of course, these abbreviations are used for convenience, too. One actual version of Leu-enkephalin with a "right-handed" alanine in that position is [D-Ala²]-Leu-enkephalin, or:

Tyr-[D-Ala]-Gly-Phe-Leu

Another, which in addition has a right-handed leucine, is [D-Ala², D-Leu⁵]-enkephalin, or:

Tyr-[D-Ala]-Gly-Phe-[D-Leu]

Another way of depicting chemical compounds, especially smaller ones like amino acids, is with a schematic drawing. Since amino acids have three-dimensional structures, depicting them this way means they get "flatted out." While a drawing doesn't give the true three-dimensionality of the molecule, it does show something the shorthand version does not: it suggests that the molecule isn't just atoms in a straight line. Parts of it do stick out here and there.

Tyrosine is made of twenty-two atoms, and it's just one of five amino acids in Leu-enkephalin. Glycine has ten atoms, and there are two glycines in both Leu- and Met-enkephalin. Leucine has twenty-two atoms in it, phenylalanine twenty-three and methionine twenty. All of which means that, including the two terminals, Leu-enkephalin has a total of ninety-four atoms, and Met-enkephalin a total of ninety-two.

Both peptides *could* be written out in the basic chemical shorthand shown in Chapter 1, the way water is written out as H_2O, but the formula so written, with more than ninety atoms in different combinations, would be terribly unwieldly. We could also depict them in illustrative schematics. But again, it would be an extremely complex drawing and hard to figure out. The easiest way—and the simplest—is to use the written shorthand of amino acid abbreviations. And the enkephalins are positively puny compared to the dynorphins, the endorphins and all their respective precursors!

Locations. The location or distribution of enkephalin-containing brain neurons is different from that of the endorphins. Using special staining techniques, scientists have found cells containing enkephalins to be widespread in the CNS. Some of the areas in which they've been found include the spinal cord and *substantia gelatinosa;* brainstem; hippocampus; *corpus striatum* and *globus pallidus;* and the central nucleus of the amygdala.

The *substantia gelatinosa* is the gray matter in the spinal cord which surrounds the cord's central canal. This is where the nerve fibers carrying information from the peripheral to the central nervous system terminate. The substantia gelatinosa is thought to be involved in modulating the transmission of pain information. A September 1981 report by British researcher J. V. Priestly noted that in the substantia gelatinosa both enkephalins and Substance P, the pain neurotransmitter, seemed to be located together in synaptic terminals.

The *globus pallidus* is part of the *lenticular nucleus,* an egg-shaped mass of gray matter which lies at the heart of the *basal ganglia.* The basal ganglia constitute the system that helps handle physical movements by passing on information from the cerebral cortex to the cerebellum and the brainstem. The *corpus striatum* is another gray matter structure often associated with the basal ganglia. Both regions, the globus pallidus and the corpus striatum, are almost literally soaked in enkephalins. The globus pallidus is packed with enkephalin-containing neuronal fibers and terminals. This area, by the way, contains no chemically detectable endorphin.

The hippocampus is an area with large concentrations of opiate receptors. It also has large concentrations of enkephalins. The central nucleus of the amygdala is also rich in enkephalins. The hippocampus is a part of the brain which is involved with emotions, learning and recognition of familiar objects. The amygdala is also a major center for emotional control. Both are part of the limbic system, the "old mammalian brain"—that wishbone-shaped "mini-brain" that is so involved in the generation and modulation of emotions.

Enkephalins, and enkephalin-containing opioid compounds, have also been found outside the CNS, most importantly in the adrenal medulla, the core of the adrenal glands. These glands sit on top of the kidneys and are the source of manufacture of several important hormones and hormonal neuromodulators, particularly epinephrine. A type of cell in the adrenal medulla called *chromaffin cell* contains within itself structures called *chromaffin granules.* These granules are important sources of enkephalin-containing peptides. Enkephalins have also been found in tumors (usually benign) of these chromaffin cells, and in other parts of the human *sympathoadrenal system,* the complex of sympathetic nerves and adrenal glands.

Alvin Stern of the Department of Molecular Genetics, Hoffman-LaRoche, in New Jersey, and several colleagues have found enkephalins in the pancreas of guinea pigs. The peptides they found there included Met- and Leu-enkephalin, and peptides six, seven and eight amino acids long that clearly came from proenkephalin, the enkephalin precursor protein. Finally, in January 1983, a group of West German researchers announced finding evidence of enkephalins in the heart. Enkephalins aren't present *everywhere* in the body, but they certainly are cropping up in a lot of different locations.

Since most of the work on enkephalins (and the other opioid peptides) has been in creatures other than humans, we also know that these chemicals are distributed widely in the animal kingdom. Humans, rats, cats, guinea pigs, sheep, cattle—all have enkephalins in their brains and bodies. Furthermore, in 1981, Floyd Bloom—then with the Salk Institute and now director of the Division of Preclinical Neuroscience and Endocrinology at the Research Institute of Scripps Clinic at La Jolla—and several colleagues found that enkephalins weren't limited to animals with backbones. They found the pentapeptides in the retinal and eyestalk neurons of lobsters. Invertebrate animals like lobsters have been around for a long time. The trilobite, distant relative to the dinner you had at that fine restaurant last week, was crawling about the ocean floor more than 500 million years ago. Of course, we don't know if trilobites had enkephalins in their eyes. But their cousins certainly do, and that says something interesting about the age and usefulness of enkephalins.

Beta-Endorphin

Discovery. The opioid peptides properly called endorphins were discovered shortly after the enkephalins. The discovery announcement by Avram Goldstein, in May 1975, did not specifically name them, though. Goldstein and his associates reported, in two separate papers, finding two different opioid peptides that were similar to, yet different from, the ones found by John Hughes and company. Neither team had characterized either compound at the time: that is, they knew they had something previously unknown, but didn't yet know the compounds' precise composition. It was, however, apparent that Goldstein's peptides were different from Hughes's and that they demonstrated opiate activity.

At the beginning of 1976, Roger Guillemin and several colleagues at the Salk Institute announced the discovery and sequencing of *alpha-endorphin*. It was a fragment of beta-lipotropin, from positions 61 to 76, and had opiate activity. There were, however, still other peptides that had not yet been identified, so Guillemin, Ling and Burgus continued their work.

At the Hormone Research Laboratory of UCSF, C. H. Li and associate David Chung came up with a peptide thirty-one amino acids long. They saw that it was identical to the sequence of thirty-one amino acids at the carboxyl terminal of his very own beta-lipotropin. This new peptide also had considerable opiate activity. Li and Chung made a synthetic version of the peptide, tested it and found it had opiate activity almost identical to the natural fragment. They suggested this new peptide be called *beta-endorphine*. The final "e" soon got dropped, and the name became beta-endorphin.

At the Addiction Research Foundation in Palo Alto, California, Avram Goldstein was quite aware of what was happening and had a good idea now of what his first 1975 peptide was. Together with Li, he quickly confirmed beta-endorphin's strong opiate activity.

In August 1976, Roger Guillemin and his associates announced the identification of a third peptide which they named *gamma-endorphin*. This new peptide actually turned out to be alpha-endorphin with one more amino acid, and was identical to the amino acids in positions 61 to 77 of beta-lipotropin.

Composition and structure. Beta-endorphin is identical to the last thirty-one amino acids in beta-lipotropin, and alpha- and gamma-endorphin are merely smaller fragments of beta-endorphin. Like the enkephalins, the endorphins begin with the amino acid sequence Tyr-Gly-Gly-Phe, which Goldstein has identified as the opiate activity message of the opioid peptides. What's more, the initial amino acid is tyrosine, with its basic nitrogen, amine-bonding property and tyramine-like structure making it oh-so-familiar to the smaller opiate alkaloid drugs. Thus the endorphins, like the drugs, are able to fit into the opiate receptors. The address part of the endorphins, positions 5 to 16 (alpha-), 17 (gamma-), or 31 (beta-), tells the molecule it can plug into either the delta or the two mu receptors. It does not seem to bind with the kappa or sigma opiate receptors.

Though synthetic versions have been made by scientists in the laboratory, the versions of Met- and Leu-enkephalin originally identified by Hughes and Kosterlitz in 1975 are the only ones found in Nature. From lobster eyestalks to human pituitaries, it's the same quintuple sequence of tyrosine, glycine, phenylalanine and either leucine or methionine.

This is not the case with beta-endorphin. C. H. Li has sequenced the beta-endorphin from at least nine different creatures—camels, cattle, sheep, pigs, horses, rats, turkeys, ostriches and salmon—and in humans. In camels, pigs and cattle the beta-endorphin is the same; in the rest it differs in some way, and in all of them it differs in some respects from human beta-endorphin. With the exception of salmon beta-endorphin, a total of eleven amino acid positions in eight different, naturally occurring molecules differ from the human norm. In salmon beta-endorphin, fully 50 percent of the amino acids differ. Four of the amino acids in salmon beta-endorphin are still not known; the molecule also seems to be two positions longer than the norm.

Distribution. Neuropharmacologists go about determining the distribution of these chemicals in the brain by using a kind of staining procedure. The process is somewhat complex, but it basically involves creating an antiserum which is sensitive to the particular peptide the researcher is looking for.

The antiserum is made in pretty much the same way any antiserum is made. Suppose what is wanted is an antiserum sensitive to the presence of beta-endorphin. First the researcher will chemically couple beta-endorphin molecules to a chemical like bovine serum albumin, a protein found in the blood of cattle. The combination, when injected into the body of an animal like a rabbit, will function as an *antigen*—it will cause the rabbit's immune system to make antibodies to fight this "invading foreign substance." Our bodies do the same thing when invaded by disease-causing bacteria.

Now the researcher removes some of the rabbit's blood, which contains antibodies to the beta-endorphin/serum albumin antigen, and removes the antibodies. These, combined with a neutral supporting fluid, comprise the beta-endorphin antiserum. When it's placed on tissue samples containing beta-endorphin, it will react with and bind to the peptide, in a manner similar to the way the rabbit antibodies earlier attacked the injected beta-endorphin/serum albumin. The researcher then washes the tissue sample. The antiserum which didn't bind is removed, leaving behind discrete areas stained with the antiserum. These areas will glow when exposed to a fluorescent light, and will shine out quite clearly in the microscope or in a micrograph.

The trick is to make an antiserum that reacts *only* to a specific peptide. An antiserum that binds to both beta-endorphin and Leu-enkephalin is not helpful when the researcher wants to determine the distribution patterns of just one of those two peptides. However, researchers have had great success in constructing antisera that are specific for the particular peptide they want to study. Specificities of 90 to 99 percent or better are no longer uncommon.

The distribution of beta-endorphin in the brain is considerably different from that of the enkephalins. At first it was thought that, since the first five amino acids in beta-endorphin and in Met-enkephalin were identical, the latter was a by-product of the former, and the enkephalins and endorphins would have similar distribution patterns. Both conclusions were wrong.

Floyd Bloom and six colleagues (Elena Battenberg, Jean Rossier, Nick Ling, Juhani Lappaluoto, Therese Vargo and Roger Guillemin) were able in 1977 to show in which particular sections of the pituitary gland two types of endorphins lay. Some researchers had at first thought alpha- and beta-endorphin were to be found in the posterior lobe of the pituitary, or perhaps throughout that gland. Bloom and his colleagues, though, using the above-described "immunofluorescence" technique, showed the two endorphins were actually present only in the intermediate *(pars intermedia)* and anterior lobes of the pituitary.

Techniques of this kind also show that the endorphin system in the brain is quite different from the enkephalin system. The enkephalins can be found in many different places in the brain: brainstem, medulla, hippocampus, corpus striatum, amygdala and other regions. The endorphins seem to be in a limited but well-defined pathway. Cell bodies in the ventral hypothalamus give rise to neuronal fibers that sweep into the preoptic region of the hypothalamus, and then on to the periaqueductal region and the pons. Endorphin-containing fibers exist in parts of the thalamus and in the periaqueductal gray, a region of the brain heavily involved in the pain transmission system. These regions stain heavily and fluoresce brightly when exposed to endorphin-specific antisera. The parts of the brain known to contain enkephalins, though, have never shown any evidence of endorphin-specific staining. Also, the enkephalin regions tend to show up as discrete dots of fluorescing stain. The endorphin regions, though, show up as definite streaks, pathways or fibers.

Endorphins, like the enkephalins, have also been found outside the brain and central nervous system. Parts of the body where they've been located include eye tissue; the pancreas; the gut; the adrenal gland; and human blood plasma. Some researchers say they've found endorphins in the human placenta, suggesting a role of endorphins in pregnancy and birth. Other researchers, though, have found evidence that the "endorphin" was actually a fragment of another compound called immunoglobin-G. It happened to have the same structure as endorphin, but wasn't the peptide at all.

Another aspect of "distribution" is the appearance of endorphins in species other than *Homo sapiens*. We've already mentioned some of them: horses, camels, cattle, sheep, pigs, rats, ostriches, turkeys, and salmon. That may seem like a wide distribution, but it covers just three classes of animals (mammals, birds, bony fishes). Beta-endorphin-like and ACTH-like material has until recently been found only in animals with pituitary and adrenal glands. These organs appeared early in the evolution of vertebrate animals, about 400 million years ago. Evolutionarily speaking, that covers only about 20 percent of the time life has existed on earth.

Some scientists have found enkephalin in the retina and eyestalk neurons of lobsters—an invertebrate animal that's a lot older on the evolutionary time scale than bony fishes like salmon. Two years ago, though, seven scientists including opiate receptor co-discoverer Candace Pert pushed the evolutionary age of endogenous opiates way back. They found beta-endorphin- and ACTH-like material in a one-celled protozoan (the proper term for these critters is "eukaryote") named *Tetrahymena pyriformis*. Creatures like *Tetrahymena* have been around for about a billion years.

Just what function these beta-endorphin-like and ACTH-like chemicals have in one-celled creatures is still not known. However, Pert and the others have also found other peptides in protozoans, peptides similar to insulin and somatostatin which resemble peptide hormones in vertebrate animals. All this suggests that these tiny, ancient one-celled beings have a gene or

genes which code for common precursors to these chemicals, and
that these genes are similar to the ones in more complex creatures like cows, pigs, camels—and people. Very early in the evolutionary history of life, then, the DNA codes for opioid peptides,
and the peptides themselves, proved useful for something. And
one of Mother Nature's most durable rules has always been: as
long as it stays useful, use it.

Dynorphin

Discovery. Kenji Kangawa and Hisayuki Matsuo of the Miyazaki
Medical College, with Masao Igarashi of the Gunma University
School of Medicine, found *alpha-neo-endorphin,* the third new endogenous opioid peptide. Their choice of a name is really somewhat unfortunate. Only in the broadest sense is it the first ("alpha") of a new ("neo") set of "endorphins." It's actually the first
of a new "genus" of endogenous opioid peptides: the *dynorphins.*
  Dynorphin itself was first isolated by Avram Goldstein and his
colleagues at the Addiction Research Foundation in Palo Alto,
California. He made the initial announcement in May 1975 at the
annual meeting of the International Narcotic Research Club—the
same meeting at which he announced the discovery of the peptide which a few months later was shown to be beta-endorphin.
But science can be like a jigsaw puzzle; sometimes the pieces
come together quickly, sometimes they don't. The discovery and
characterization of the endorphins unfolded quickly, in a matter
of months. Dynorphin was the other side of the coin. It took more
than four years for Goldstein to finally be able to characterize it as
something really different from the enkephalins and the endorphins.
  Goldstein and his team began their ultimately successful experiment to determine the nature of "slow-reversing endorphin"
with a hundred grams of melanotropin concentrate from pig
pituitary glands. (Melanotropin is a hormone that in humans
regulates skin color.) A hundred grams is about three and a half
ounces, the weight of two golf balls. After a long process of

filtration and purification, they ended up with the equivalent of a few micrograms of pure peptide. A microgram is a millionth of a gram, in this case a hundred-millionth of what they started with. Take those two golf balls, chop them each up into fifty million pieces, and then throw away all but one piece. You're left with very little.

Goldstein and S. Tachibana, Louise Downey, Michael Hunkapiller and Leroy Hood determined the sequence of the first thirteen amino acids in his peptide, and the latter's potency. It was very powerful. In the standard test of opiate potency, the guinea pig ileum test, Goldstein's peptide was seven hundred times as potent as Leu-enkephalin, two hundred times as powerful as morphine and fifty times as powerful as camel beta-endorphin. A mere eighty micrograms of the peptides injected into the lateral ventricle of rats sent the little animals into almost immediate catalepsy and analgesia. Goldstein named the peptide *dynorphin*, from the Greek prefix "dyn-" (meaning power). It was also referred to as "dynorphin-13," for the number of amino acids so far known to be in it.

Later Goldstein identified the rest of the molecule. It turned out to have seventeen amino acids in it; the last four didn't seem to add to its potency. Goldstein and other researchers then found other dynorphins of other sizes, including dynorphin-8 (a fragment), dynorphin-24, -32 and -B, and in July of 1982 the dynorphin precursor, pre-prodynorphin. It contained all the dynorphin peptides as well as the alpha-neo-endorphin sequence. This last turned out to be beta-neo-endorphin plus the lysine of the lysine-arginine processing signal which followed it. So it's probably simplest to just call it "neo-endorphin."

Composition and structure. Dynorphin is a Leu-enkephalin-containing opioid peptide which shows immense opiate activity in the standard tests for such things. The smallest complete molecule, dynorphin-17, begins with the Leu-enkephalin sequence and is followed by twelve additional amino acids. Dynorphin-24 includes dynorphin-17 followed by Lys-Arg (the amino acids lysine and arginine). Then there follows a second Leu-enkephalin sequence. Dynorphin-32 has all this followed by two arginines (Arg-Arg) and six additional amino acids. Dynorphin[20-32], beginning with the second Leu-enkephalin sequence, is another dynorphin peptide which like the others has been found in living tissue. Goldstein named it dynorphin-B. Sid Udenfriend has called it rimorphin. Neo-endorphin is a peptide nine amino acids long, resembling in some ways the other dynorphin peptides. It begins with a Leu-enkephalin sequence and is followed by four additional amino acids. Neo-endorphin [6-7] is arginine and lysine, which Goldstein calls a processing signal. In this instance, though, it may not function as a processing signal.

All these compounds are found within pre-prodynorphin, the dynorphin/neo-endorphin precursor. All but one are flanked on either side by the processing signals Lys-Arg or Arg-Arg. The one exception is the dynorphin-32 sequence. It's a little puzzling. It does *not* end with a standard processing signal, but with Arg-Ser, or arginine and serine. Has someone made a mistake? Is it possible dynorphin-32 is a fragment of some much longer peptide, one which runs past the end of the known pre-prodynorphin sequence and into the still undeciphered nucleotide tail? Well, it's possible, all right. However, Udenfriend and company have found dynorphin[20-32] (dynorphin-B) in living brain tissue. So it is being created there; peptidases do break the precursor at its position 240, at the Arg-Ser duo. This is the only known instance in the opioid peptides where that duo serves as a cleavage site.

The discoverers of dynorphin were naturally intrigued by the astounding potency of this peptide, and wondered which amino acids in which positions might be specifically responsible for it. Goldstein's colleague Charles Chavkin removed one amino acid at a time from the C-terminal of dynorphin-13 and found out. The —COOH itself was not important to opiate power. Removing the lysine at position 13 (called Lys[13]) did cause a slight drop in potency, but Chavkin found it was caused by the —COOH interfering chemically with Leu[12]. Chopping Leu[12] off restored dynorphin to nearly full power. However, when Chavkin then removed the lysine at position 11, he found that what was left— dynorphin[1-10]—had very little opiate potency. Another major drop happened when he removed Arg[7]. Those two amino acids in dynorphin, the arginine at position 7 and the lysine at position 11, are essential to the incredible power of dynorphin.

The reason, Goldstein hypothesizes, lies in the construction of the dynorphin receptor, the kappa receptor. Goldstein thinks that the "message" part of dynorphin, the "Tyr-Gly-Gly-Phe" part at the beginning which says "this chemical will initiate opiate-like activity," fits into a pocket in the kappa receptor. Since all the opioid peptides begin with that fourfold sequence, that pocket is similar to the ones in the other opiate receptors. The kappa receptor, though, has two additional pockets which accommodate the electrical charges on arginine at position 7 and lysine at position 11 in the "address" portion of dynorphin. This makes it possible for dynorphin to fit into the kappa receptor; those two pockets, when filled by those two specific amino acids at those two positions, will also signal a manyfold increase in opiate potency.

Interestingly enough, both dynorphin-B and neo-endorphin also seem to interact with the kappa receptor, and the latter is possessed of considerable opiate potency. Dynorphin-B has an arginine at its position 7, as does dynorphin-17 or -A, but a valine at position 11. Dynorphin-B is known to be weaker in opiate potency than dynorphin-A. Neo-endorphin has a lysine at its position 7. However, lysine and arginine have similar structures —they are the only two amino acids with open carbon chains, one —COOH radical and two NH_2— radicals—and their DNA codes are similar. Neo-endorphin has no position 11, but the great similarity between arginine and lysine must certainly be part of the explanation for its potent opiate activity via the dynorphin receptor.

Distribution. Goldstein and other researchers have tracked down the distribution of dynorphin in the central nervous system by using a particularly good radioimmunoassay, or RIA. In some ways similar to the immunofluorescent technique that Floyd Bloom first used to distinguish the endorphin and enkephalin neuropathways, RIA uses hormones and antibodies that are radioactively tagged rather than fluorescently tagged. It's an extremely sensitive method, and can spot concentrations of proteins as small as a few trillionths of a gram (called a picogram). Remember that piece of golf ball weighing a few micrograms? A picogram is a million times smaller.

Goldstein developed an antiserum called "Lucia" which was extremely specific for dynorphin in RIA tests. It did not get confused by Leu-enkephalin, even though dynorphin-17 and -B have a Leu-enkephalin sequence at their beginnings and dynorphin-24 and -32 have two of them. It is also not fooled by neo-endorphin; as the scientists would phrase it, Lucia "cross-reacts" with neo-endorphin only at about one ten-thousandth of a percent.

Using the Lucia antiserum (and other techniques as well), brain researchers have found dynorphin in many places in the body. Dynorphin in the pituitary gland is almost entirely in the posterior portion. The posterior lobe of pig pituitaries, for example, had 97 percent of all the pituitary's dynorphin. This is similar to the enkephalin concentration in the pituitary, which is also predominantly in the posterior lobe. However, beta-endorphin doesn't appear in that part of the pituitary at all; it's found mainly in the anterior lobe and the pars intermedia.

Dynorphin exists in other parts of the brain as well. Nearly a third of the total dynorphin in the brain is in the cortex; the medulla and the pons have another 20 percent. It had also been found in high concentrations in the supraoptic nucleus, which is part of the hypothalamus; in the medulla and pons at the bottom of the brain; and in the cerebellum. The rear hypothalamus has the highest concentration of dynorphin; it is followed, in diminishing order of concentration, by the front hypothalamus; the medulla, pons and midbrain; the hippocampus; striatum; cortex; and cerebellum. This differs from the enkephalin concentration pattern in the brain; enkephalin is most highly concentrated in the striatum. The dynorphin concentration pattern also differs from that of beta-endorphin, which is almost completely absent from the striatum, hippocampus, cerebellum and cortex.

There are also high concentrations of dynorphin in the spinal cord. The highest concentrations are in the dorsal or rear part of the cord, followed by somewhat lower dynorphin concentrations in the ventral (front) cord and in the dorsal horn of the spinal cord. The dorsal cord, it turns out, is very important to the body's pain sensation system. So dynorphin is shown to be involved in the transmission of information related to pain. Dynorphin has also been found in the nerve networks serving parts of the guinea pig small intestine. In late 1980, Charles Chavkin and Avram Goldstein showed that this nerve network—the myenteric plexus —which is used in tests of opiate potency, contained the specific dynorphin receptor, the kappa receptor.

Floyd Bloom had several years earlier shown that the central nervous system had separate endorphin- and enkephalin-containing systems. Now Goldstein and other researchers had demonstrated that dynorphin made up a third system, separate from that of both beta-endorphin and the enkephalins. By contrast, the distribution of neo-endorphin turned out to be remarkably similar to that of dynorphin. In fact, the two are almost completely identical.

Leading the way to this discovery were Eckard Weber, Kevin Roth and Jack Barchas of Stanford University. They used antisera to both dynorphin and neo-endorphin in immunofluorescent studies. The dynorphin antiserum didn't react with neo-endorphin, and vice versa. Neither of them reacted with Leu-enkephalin, either, so there was no chance of that throwing the results off. Weber, Roth and Barchas would first stain a slice of rat brain with one antiserum, and photograph the results under fluorescent light. Then they'd remove the first antiserum from the tissue, stain it with the other, and photograph the tissue again. They found the same places in the tissue stained with both antisera. In fact, the photographs were totally superimposable. One phototransparency could be laid over the other, and the stain patterns would be identical. All the places that were known to have dynorphin-containing nerve fibers— parts of the hypothalamus, the medulla, the *substantia nigra* in the brainstem, the hippocampus and others—also had neo-endorphin. They found no place that had either of the two peptides alone.

The three Stanford researchers also found that parts of the dynorphin/neo-endorphin system at least partly overlapped the enkephalin system. Leu-enkephalin turned out to be present in some nerve pathways which contained dynorphin and neo-endorphin. So it's at least possible there's some kind of partial connection between those two systems. For example, there may be some circumstances in which Leu-enkephalin does get cleaved from dynorphin or neo-endorphin. The amino acid processing signals Arg-Lys, Lys-Arg and/or Arg-Arg flank all three Leu-enkephalin sequences in pre-prodynorphin.

Weber and Barchas, along with Christopher Evans, have made another interesting discovery about the distribution of dynorphin and alpha-neo-endorphin. In many of the brain regions containing the two peptides, neo-endorphin has seemed to be present in much higher quantities than dynorphin. It now turns out that these areas actually have concentrations of a dynorphin fragment, dynorphin-8, the first eight amino acids in the peptide.

Dynorphin-8 is only about 3 percent as powerful as dynorphin-17, but the brain has ten times as much dynorphin-8 as it does dynorphin-17. What's more, Weber and company have found dynorphin-8 and neo-endorphin in equimolar concentrations everywhere in the brain they've looked.

This means we may have to reexamine the function of dynorphin-17 in the central nervous system. There's only twice as much dynorphin-8 as dynorphin-17 in the spinal cord, but ten times as much in parts of the brain such as the striatum and midbrain regions. Apparently some neurons break dynorphin down more completely in some places than in others. The neurons in the dorsal cord area of the spine, for example, may well need relatively large amounts of dynorphin-17 for its high opiate potency, since this is a part of the CNS that transmits and modifies pain signals. Other areas of the nervous system, though, don't need potent dynorphin, so they break dynorphin-17 down to dynorphin-8.

Finally, we must say something about *Bufo marinus. Bufo marinus* is a species of toad. Just as enkephalins and endorphins have been found in creatures other than mammals (enkephalins as far down the evolutionary scale as lobsters, for example, and endorphins in primitive one-celled protozoans), so dynorphin is not limited in species distribution to rats, guinea pigs and people. Ric Cone and Avram Goldstein have found dynorphins in toads. They used an antiserum sensitive to pig dynorphin, so it's likely that toad dynorphin is nearly identical in structure to pig dynorphin. That would make sense; we've already seen that ostrich beta-endorphin (class: birds) is 80 percent identical to pig beta-endorphin (class: mammals). And more than that: Goldstein and Cone found three different kinds of dynorphin in *Bufo,* and that eventually led to the discovery of dynorphin-24 and dynorphin-32. So hurray for *Bufo* the toad, who gave his spinal cord, brain and pituitary gland for science.

*   *   *

Most of the major work determining the biochemical nature, structure and origins of the three known "genera" of endogenous opioid peptides has been done. We know what the endorphins are made of, where they are made and how they are made. We know a lot about their family tree, since we have found the protein precursors and have learned something about the process from precursor to final peptide.

Many questions remain to be answered. We don't know all the details about the biosynthetic pathways of the opioid peptides, how they proceed from DNA code through precursor protein to final form. There are a lot of intermediate-sized enkephalin-containing peptides (ECPs) floating around in the body, too. What functions, if any, do they have? The dynorphin/enkephalin connection is still puzzling, too. Are the dynorphins and/or the dynorphin precursor sources of Leu-enkephalin? Is that why the dynorphin and enkephalin pathways in the brain overlap in some places? The questions go on and on.

Nevertheless, we have learned a lot about the endorphins in the years since their initial discovery. And we have begun to learn a little about what they may do in living creatures. Including us. In the next five chapters we'll take a look at some of the things endorphins may do.

PART II

THE CONNECTIONS

6

Endorphins and Pain

A home on Goldcrest Heights. During the day Mt. Rainier's shattered cone is visible from the front window. But not at 2 A.M.

Why is it that babies insist on being born at 2 A.M.? Tiffany wonders. They don't always, but at this time of the morning she remembers only the babies born in the still of the night. Tiffany is a midwife, 2004-style. Much has changed in the twenty-one years since she was born. Then, her profession was just beginning to emerge from a long twilight of ignorance and neglect. Most babies were still born in hospitals and most mothers still had their spines soaked in opiate-based drugs that may have deadened the pain of childbirth but also threatened the health of the infant.

Not now. Genna puffs furiously and Peter puffs with her. Off in a corner a friend is timing the contractions. They're getting closer. Tiffany leans over her charge. "Gen, we're going to give you the injection now," she says gently. "It's not going to hurt, just sting a little." She and Peter help the woman roll partly onto her right side. Out of the traditional black bag comes a syringe and a rubber-topped vial. In and out: the syringe is filled. Quickly, deftly, Tiffany administers an injection of Genna's own beta-endorphin (removed from her body two weeks earlier) into her lower spine.

* * *

When researchers began doing experiments with endorphins and enkephalins, one of the first things they poked at was the possible connection between these chemicals and the way we experience pain. There was a good reason for that. The opioid peptides had been discovered in the first place because of their great similarity to drugs like morphine, the classic pain-killer. If an externally produced drug like morphine was so effective at suppressing pain in humans (and other animals), perhaps endorphins did the same thing naturally. Neurobiologists and neuropharmacologists grabbed a bunch of experimental rats and dashed off to their labs.

But first things first: What *is* pain?

Defining Pain

One definition of pain is that it's "an unpleasant experience which we associate with tissue damage, or describe in terms of such damage, or both." The phrase "unpleasant experience" is pretty subjective for something that's supposed to be an objective scientific definition.

But pain is, in essence, a subjective thing. We can never directly perceive each other's pain. The actual *experience* that each person undergoes is forever locked into her or his own mind. No other human can ever fully know or understand the pain *you* feel.

Pain is also a sensory experience unlike others. Like sight or hearing, for example, it involves the transmission of information from "the outside world" to the central nervous system; unlike those senses, however, pain produces an experience that leads us to engage in behavior to stop the pain. An experience often resulting from pain is one we call "suffering."

But suffering and pain are not always connected to each other. Sometimes people experience pain but are not distressed by it. And psychological sensations and experiences unconnected to physical damage or disease can lead to the experience of distress or suffering.

Though the pain and suffering each of us experiences is ultimately subjective, we all assume from shared information about our sensory experiences that the experiences are common to us all. This includes pain and suffering. We can "empathize" with another's pain. We also assume that animals' experience of pain is similar to ours. But because pain *is* such a subjective experience, it's important to recognize these assumptions we're making. This is especially true when we talk about the connections between the experience of pain and suffering on the one hand and the operations of chemicals like beta-endorphin and dynorphin on the other. For the subjective experience of pain has powerful objective connections to physical and chemical processes.

The Process of "Ouch!"

How does the pain system work? Well, suppose you've been trying to whittle. You used to do it as a kid, but that was a long time ago. You're older now and should know better than to try and recapture your scouting days. But out comes the old Swiss army knife, and you start in on a piece of broken chair leg.

And almost at once slice into your left thumb.

The process begins with the activation of sensors in your thumb. These are "free nerve endings"; they're just hanging out there at the edge of your body, the surface of your skin. Several different kinds of receptors report sensations which are interpreted as pain. Some are fixed-response receptors: they respond only to heat and cold, for example. Others are multiple-response receptors, with the capability of signaling in response to a variety of different stimuli.

Not all stimuli are unpleasant in themselves. But some receptors, called *nociceptors*, respond only to stimuli that are rightly called "noxious"—a truly extreme change in temperature (you just brushed the hot stove burner with your elbow), or a massive dislocation of internal organs and bones (you're nine years old and you just fell off the top of the jungle gym and broke your right leg).

The cut in your thumb is detected by a mixture of these different kinds of sensors, and it's a mixture of impulses that goes racing down the nerves, jumping synapses and heading for your brain.

The impulses head off along at least two different nerve paths. One, called the "A-Delta nerves," is the "fast pain" route. The message traveling over this route will be the first to reach the brain, with the report that dum-dum did something to the left thumb. The second nerve path, the "C fibers," as they're called, carries a more continuous message to the brain. This is the message that the brain will probably translate as that "aching feeling" in your left thumb.

The first message thus signals the brain: "Alert! Something's wrong in the left thumb!" The second message, coming through the C fibers, tells the brain that the noxious stimulus called "a cut in the skin and muscle of the left thumb" is there—it's still there, better do something about it—it's still there, do something—it's still there, better do something—until you do something.

These particular sets of A-Delta fibers and C fibers go up through the hand and arm and then eventually into the spinal cord. They enter the cord in places called the *dorsal* and *ventral roots,* and in the *dorsal horn* region. This part of the spinal cord is a very important part of the nociceptive (pain transmission) system.

The dorsal horn (or dorsal cord) is a rearward projection of gray matter of the spinal cord. It's here that the signals from your thumb arrive, and it's here that they can be modified by signals from other nerve receptors. Signals coming down from your brain can modify the pain stimulus. If you are in a mental state called hypnosis or are meditating when you cut your thumb, your brain may be sending signals down to the dorsal horn to modify the pain stimulus. That modification can also happen in the brain itself.

If the signal isn't totally suppressed, it continues up the spinal cord to the brain via two separate pathways or tracts. One is called the *spinothalamic tract.* It runs up the spinal cord and into the thalamus. The thalamus is the part of the brainstem that functions as the receiving, associating and synthesizing center for every sense except smell. Here is where the other sensory perceptions connected with your cutting your finger get blended together: the pressure of the knife blade; the sight of the blood spurting out; the feel of the blood running out onto your thumb and hand; the tightening sense of your muscles jerking as you automatically react to the damage to your thumb; the sound of your own startled voice crying out in anger. From the thalamus a whole network of nerves and neurons radiates into the cerebral cortex. And as you experience what you've done, you at once begin understanding and intellectualizing what you've done.

The spinothalamic tract is the more direct route to the brain for pain sensations. The second pathway, the *spinoreticular tract,* is slower. "Reticular" means meshed or like a network, and that's what this pathway is: a more diffuse network of nerves that carry the pain signal to the brain. This tract relays the pain stimuli to several small masses of gray matter that are buried deep in the brain's hemispheres. Two of them are known collectively as the *corpus striatum.* From here the pain sensations are relayed to other areas in the brain, places like the hippocampus and the *cingulate gyrus.* These are parts of the brain connected with motivational and emotional behavior, and with memory.

It's not too surprising that the pain sensations end up in such places in the brain. Pain, like pleasure, is a great motivator. In fact, that might be its evolutionary function. Pleasure motivates a creature to do things that are pro-survival; pain motivates it to avoid things that are anti-survival.

In your case, you are motivated to do something about the cut thumb. You head for the medicine cabinet. You may also use your reasoning process to decide you'll be a bit more careful the next time you try to whittle a broken chair leg.

The endorphins play an important role in this process of nociception. Researchers have found beta-endorphin, enkephalins and dynorphins in many of the regions we've just looked at, including the spinal cord's dorsal horn and the corpus striatum. They've also been found in another area of the brain important to pain perception. It's called the *nucleus raphe magnus.* The nucleus raphe magnus is a small group of neurons at the bottom rear of the brain, near two of the small cavities or ventricles of the brain. Neurons in the raphe magnus have long axons extending down into the dorsal horn at various levels of the spinal column. We've already seen how the dorsal horn is an area where pain signals can be modified by signals from other senses.

The raphe magnus doesn't sit in isolation in the brain, though. Just above it in the brain, surrounding a narrow canal that drains brain fluid into the spinal column, is a layer of gray matter called the *periaqueductal gray* ("gray matter surrounding the aqueduct" is a literal translation). The periaqueductal gray (often abbreviated PAG) is practically saturated with endorphins. And it has axons that extend down into the raphe magnus.

So the PAG is connected to the raphe magnus (RM), and the raphe magnus is connected to the dorsal horn (DH), and the dorsal horn is where pain signals are modified or suppressed on their way up to the brain via the spinoreticular tract.

Are we beginning to see the connection? The researchers do. They believe that endorphins, known to be similar to pain-killers like morphine in their chemical structure, operate in this "PG-to-RM-to-DH" pathway to inhibit pain signals.

The Endorphin/Pain Connection

Researchers began finding connections between endogenous peptides and pain almost as soon as they discovered the peptides. In 1976 two separate teams of scientists—one group working for Wyeth Laboratories in Philadelphia, the other for the Sandoz drug company in Switzerland—injected Met-enkephalin and Leu-enkephalin into the brains of mice and rats. They quickly found that both enkephalins had analgesic effects under those circumstances. They also discovered that they could cancel or reverse the pain-killing effects of the enkephalins by first injecting the animals with doses of naloxone, the drug used to counteract the effects of morphine and heroin. Enkephalin had a pain-killing effect much weaker than morphine or heroin, and it didn't last nearly as long—but in other ways the endogenous peptide acted much like its more well-known chemical cousins.

The Sandoz researchers also concocted a synthetic chemical that was just the first three amino acids (Tyr-Gly-Gly) of enkephalin. When they checked to see if this "tripeptide" would also have pain-killing effects similar in some way to the full enkephalin molecule, they found it didn't. In Chapter 4 we noted how the first four parts of all opioid peptides are the essential "address" for opiate receptor sites on nerves. Phe[4] and Met or Leu[5] of molecule are also essential for any analgesic effect to be present, at least when they're injected directly into the central nervous systems of mice.

However, the most surprising finding (to the researchers, anyway) of these early experiments was not that enkephalins were naturally produced pain-killers, but that it seemed to take *so much* enkephalin to produce *such a small result.* The Wyeth researchers had used doses of one hundred to two hundred micrograms of enkephalins, introduced right into the rats' brains, and had gotten only a few minutes of analgesia. The Sandoz team had used doses of enkephalins running up to more than four hundred micrograms per mouse, and gotten similarly short responses. A few hundred millionths of a gram of a substance may seem like very little; but in this case it wasn't at all. For the standard pain-killer morphine produced analgesia lasting *seven times longer* with doses ten to a hundred times *smaller.*

Meanwhile, four scientists created a synthetic enkephalin that was both a potent and a long-lasting analgesic. The team included Jaw-Kang Chang and Bosco T. W. Fong of Beckman Instruments, Inc., of Palo Alto, California, and Agu Pert and opiate receptor co-discoverer Candace Pert of the National Institute of Mental Health in Maryland. The substance they created was an *amide,* an organic molecule that has at one end the atoms $-CONH_2$ instead of the more common $-COOH$. Chang, Fong and the Perts also changed part of the enkephalin pentapeptide chain itself. They replaced the second amino acid, Gly^2, with a right-handed version of the amino acid alanine, or $D-Ala^2$. Its whole structure is $H-Tyr-[D-Ala]-Gly-Phe-Met-CONH_2$, which they called "DALA" (instead of "$[D-Ala^2]$-Met-enkephalinamide," a huge mouthful even for scientists).

When they tested the analgesic potency of this new synthetic version of Met-enkephalin, they found that only five micrograms of DALA began having analgesic properties only fifteen minutes after being injected into rats. The effects lasted for up to three hours. With ten micrograms, the rats were still showing significant pain-killing effects three hours later. Five micrograms of morphine had the same effects as ten of DALA. The clincher was that naloxone injections stopped the effects of DALA—stopped them cold, just as it affected the activity of morphine.

The secret of DALA's pain-killing potency is in the D-Ala. In regular enkephalin, the chemical bond between the first two amino acids (Tyr and Gly) is weak enough for peptidases and enkephalinases to break. That leads to the destruction of enkephalin. D-alanine is a form of alanine which is "right-handed." The "D" stands for *dexter*, the Latin word meaning "right [-handed]." It is a mirror image, as it were, of the more normal "left-handed" form of alanine. The molecule's reverse shape puts part of the amino acid's structure in a position that makes it very difficult for the enzymes to get in and break the bond between the tyrosine and the D-alanine. The whole peptide lasts longer and remains more potent. (And just as an aside: when "normal" L-Ala is substituted for Gly^2 in the enkephalinamide, it has only *one tenth* of regular enkephalin's analgesic potency. Even in Nature, it often pays to be right-handed.)

Shutting Down Substance P

Experimenters continued to explore the exciting connections between the endorphins/enkephalins and the pain process. In 1977 two researchers in Great Britain, Leslie L. Iverson and T. M. Jessell, looked at how endorphins, enkephalins and morphine influenced the action of a chemical called *Substance P.*

Substance P is a peptide found in many parts of the central nervous system connected with the transmission of pain signals. It is a powerful exciter of neurons in the spinal cord and in the dorsal horn region (which we've learned is a major modification nexus for pain transmission). Substance P seems to selectively excite neurons that are specifically connected with transmitting signals of noxious stimuli. Thus Substance P (or SP) has long been considered one of the major neurotransmitters of pain signals, if not the major one.

Iverson and Jessell found that when they introduced morphine into slices of rat brainstems and spinal cords, it inhibited the release of Substance P. The effect was "dose dependent": the more morphine they added, the less SP was released. Adding naloxone just before the morphine resulted in a reversal of the morphine's effect on the SP, but adding just naloxone did nothing to the release of SP.

Then the two researchers performed the same test with DALA, and later with beta-endorphin. The two endogenous opioid peptides had the same essential effect as the morphine: *they inhibited the release of SP from the tissue slices.*

Their explanation of their findings: endogenous opiates somehow act *presynaptically* to inhibit the release of SP from the ends of neurons that are transmitting pain signals. A kind of neuron called an *interneuron* (because it's an "intermediate" neuron) has its axon coming up to the neuron which is releasing SP. Under certain conditions the interneuron will release enkephalins or beta-endorphin, which plug into opiate receptor sites on the SP-releasing neuron. This inhibits its release of Substance P, and ends up inhibiting the pain signal.

Endorphins, Pain—and People

By 1980 evidence had begun appearing that the endorphins were involved not only in the pain transmission system of rats and mice —but also in that of a high-order mammal called *Homo sapiens.*

The first report came from a team that included Nobel Prize winner Roger Guillemin of the Salk Institute in San Diego. Guillemin and associate Nicholas Ling in 1979 supplied three Japanese researchers (Tsutomu Oyama, Toshiro Jin and Ryuji Yamaya) with some of their synthetic beta-endorphin. The Japanese wanted to see if beta-endorphin would have analgesic effects on humans. They took fourteen patients with previously untreatable pain from widespread cancer and with their permission gave them injections of three milligrams of Guillemin and Ling's synthetic beta-endorphin. The injections were intrathecal (that is, into the spinal column) and not intracranial (into the head or brain).

The results were dramatic. *All fourteen of the patients received profound and long-lasting relief from pain that had formerly been impossible to control.* The relief lasted an average of 33.4 hours, and in one case for *more than three days.* The people involved were four women and ten men; their ages ranged from twenty-nine to sixty-eight. Most of them fell asleep after the beta-endorphin injection (certainly a blessing, for many had found it almost impossible to get any sleep because of their intense pain). Others experienced a euphoric feeling after getting the beta-endorphin. Three seemed to be somewhat disoriented, and two had difficulty urinating—both symptoms common with reception of opiate analgesics like morphine.

Five of the patients also got a placebo injection, to serve as a control to the effects of the endorphin. Three of them got no relief at all; the other two received placebo pain relief that lasted for only a fraction of the time of the endorphin's relief.

One of the most remarkable results of this dramatic experiment was the rapid beginning of pain relief (from one to sixteen minutes). It was a completely unexpected thing, because previous experiments with animals had suggested that the endorphins would have to be injected into the brain for the analgesic effects to begin quickly. To the five researchers the results strongly suggested that the endorphin/pain reaction takes place first *in the spinal cord,* not in the brain. Both endorphins and endorphin-type receptor sites had already been found in areas of the spine, but this was the first time anyone had found real evidence that endorphins were involved in the nociceptive system in humans, and in humans' spinal cord regions.

The five researchers also pointed out how effective beta-endorphin had been in patients who had gotten at best only partial pain relief from large and frequent doses of "normal" opiates. That seemed to suggest that the receptor sites were better-attuned to the body's own natural pain-killers—endorphins and enkephalins—than to exogenous opiate drugs.

This wasn't the only experiment with endorphins and pain in humans in 1980. Later that year, Ling, Guillemin, Oyama and two other Japanese doctors announced results of tests of synthetic human beta-endorphin in relieving the pain of childbirth in fourteen women. Here things were a bit more chancy; not only adult humans but also soon-to-be-born infants were involved.

But the results were just as dramatic as those for the cancer patients. The fourteen women received the endorphin intrathecally at the time of delivery. All fourteen got rapid and prolonged analgesia during delivery. They all had normal uterine contractions; were awake and cooperative during delivery; and had none of the symptoms of depressed breathing rate, heartbeat or central nervous functioning that can happen with opiate analgesics like morphine.

And all the babies were completely normal.

One reason was probably the placenta. Like the blood-brain barrier (or BBB), the placenta acts as a filter, keeping some chemicals from reaching the fetus. That's not all it does, of course. It's primarily doing the opposite: supplying the fetus with blood and nourishment from the mother's system. So the barrier function is not perfect. Alcohol can pass through the placenta, giving rise to the tragedy of fetal alcohol syndrome: babies with mental and physical defects caused by their mothers' drinking. Morphine, heroin and many drugs used as analgesics in childbirth can also cross the placenta into the fetus and have serious effects on it. Endorphins, though, are larger molecules. They don't seem to be able to get through the placenta. So the newborn infants showed no effects from the injections of synthetic beta-endorphin their mothers got.

The Japanese experiments showed that beta-endorphin, injected into the spinal cord of humans, had powerful analgesic effects. But Yoshio Hosobuchi, of the UCSF School of Medicine, and Guillemin, Floyd Bloom and Jean Rossier came up with the first evidence for *the actual release of beta-endorphin-like substances* in living humans.

Pain in humans can sometimes be alleviated by electrically stimulating certain parts of the brain, especially the periaqueductal gray (PAG) and nearby periventricular gray (PVG) matter. And we saw earlier that the PAG is an important part of the nociceptive system. This phenomenon is usually called "stimulation-produced analgesia," or SPA. The four scientists were able to collect cerebrospinal fluid from the brains of people undergoing SPA—before, during and after the treatment. In three patients with electrodes implanted in the PAG, the levels of beta-endorphin-like substances in the brain fluid increased *two to four times* when they got electrical stimulation to relieve their pain.

Coupled with earlier findings, that year, of pain relief from injections of beta-endorphin, this experiment has provided some of the firmest and most exciting evidence that endorphins are definitely connected with how we feel pain, and how we can stop it.

Something to Sink Your Teeth Into

A *placebo* is an inert, inactive substance that of itself is incapable of doing anything in the body—but which sometimes does have medical effects. Sugared water or pills containing some tasteless and harmless white powder are often used as analgesics with people suffering terminal illnesses. For even though the placebo itself contains nothing that can alleviate pain, a certain percentage of people will nevertheless *receive pain relief when they take it.* This is referred to as the "analgesic placebo effect," and why it even exists has been a puzzle to doctors for a long time.

The major experiment pointing to a role for endorphins in the analgesic placebo effect was performed in 1978 by three researchers at the University of California at San Francisco. Jon Levine, Newton Gordon and Howard Fields worked with fifty-one men and women suffering from impacted wisdom teeth. The subjects ranged in age from the late teens through the early thirties, and were in good health (except for the impacted wisdom teeth).

The three researchers told the patients they might receive injections of morphine, a placebo or naloxone, which counteracts morphine's pain-killing effect. The people who got naloxone could expect a possible increase in pain. All the patients gave full informed consent.

Levine et al. were attempting what's called a "double-blind" test, in which neither the subjects *nor* the researchers know who's getting what. The bottles containing the substances to be tested are labeled only with code numbers. The researchers keep track of which person (or animal) gets which dose from which coded bottle. When all have gotten whatever they're going to get, the code is broken. *Then* the researchers know who got what—but not until. In this way, researchers hope to eliminate any possibility of unconscious bias in their testing.

In this particular test, the double-blind was being partly broken. While the researchers didn't know who was going to get what (morphine, naloxone or placebo), the patients knew they were going to get *one* of the three substances. Even that is something ordinarily not revealed to patients, since such knowledge could predispose some people to certain kinds of reactions; however, the three researchers claim that previous experiments of a similar nature had not been adversely affected by the revelation of such knowledge to the patients.

After the subjects had their wisdom teeth removed (under standard anesthetics) and had spent some time in a recovery room, they each received at random two separate injections of either one or two of the three possible substances—morphine, naloxone or a placebo. They got the first injection two hours after the beginning of anesthesia for the tooth extraction. The second injection came an hour after the first.

The people who got morphine during the test were not included in the final analysis, because morphine is known to kill pain, and naloxone is known to block its effects. The point of the experiment was to find out *how naloxone affected reactions to a placebo, and vice versa.* The morphine-injected people were thus the "controls," whose reactions could be known in advance and against which the others' reactions could be compared.

Everyone also had the option of dropping out of the test before it was over, and five did, leaving forty-six men and women whose reactions to the placebo and/or naloxone were studied.

The results?

• About 40 percent of the people in the test were "placebo responders." That is, their pain ratings showed that they were reacting to the placebo as if it were a pain-killer.

• The so-called placebo responders who got naloxone as the second injection had pain ratings *higher* than those who were not placebo responders. The naloxone had no effect on the pain ratings of the nonresponders, but it brought the ratings of those who were responders up to the level of those who weren't. This suggested to the researchers that most if not all of any pain-suppressing effect produced by the placebo was being reversed by naloxone.

• Five of the fourteen (out of an initial seventeen) people who got the placebo injection both times reported a *decrease* in pain after the second placebo injection.

· Of the eleven people who received the naloxone first and the placebo second, only two reported a decrease in pain.

· All twenty-three people who got the placebo first and the naloxone second reported significantly *more* pain than did the people who got the placebo both times. That, too, strongly suggests that the naloxone was blocking the pain-suppressing action of *something* that was supposed to be *nothing.*

Naloxone, as we mentioned earlier, is used to counteract the effects of heroin and morphine. That's why it and similar chemicals are called opiate *antagonists.* And by 1978, it was well known that naloxone and its brethren also counteracted the action of the endorphins in experimental testing.

But the placebo was a, well, a *placebo!* It was neither morphine nor an endorphin. Yet the placebo responders who got naloxone injections after the placebo injections reported more pain than the people who didn't respond to the placebo. In fact, *everyone* who got the naloxone as a second injection reported pain levels higher than those who got the placebo only.

Since the morphine recipients were not included in this final analysis, Fields and Gordon and Levine had to conclude that the people who reacted as placebo responders were somehow actually producing increased levels of endorphins in their bodies, in order to counteract the pain of the tooth extractions.

Believing that what they were getting in the injection might be the pain-killer morphine, the subjects were going about producing pain-killing endorphins to do the work. But when they got the second injection of naloxone, that chemical counteracted—*antagonized*—the endorphins' pain-suppressing effect.

It was a clever experiment. It seemed to show quite clearly that the placebo effect was caused by endorphins. It's a classic case of "mind over matter," or "mind controlling matter." The people thought they were getting a pain-killer. They weren't. But they thought they were. So their bodies simply manufactured more of their natural pain-killers, endorphins, to do the job.

Unfortunately, this particular experiment has never been precisely duplicated with the same results occurring. That's a puzzle, and a serious one. The essence of the scientific method is reproducible results. Is it possible that the gap in their double-blind was not as innocuous as Fields and his colleagues thought? Possible.

One thing's certain, though. If the experiment doesn't prove a placebo/endorphin connection, it certainly makes its possibility a lot more intriguing.

Acupuncture and Endorphins

If endorphins are part of the body's system for relieving pain, then the levels of these endogenous opiates in the body should rise when pain-relieving techniques are used. One of the better-known methods is acupuncture.

In acupuncture one or more needles are inserted into specific points on the body. The free ends of the needles may be twirled about, and sometimes a weak electrical current is passed through the needles. This last version is called electroacupuncture, or EAP. The anesthesia produced has been sufficient to permit surgery without other forms of anesthesia.

Exactly how acupuncture works is still not completely known, but the evidence is pretty persuasive that it does. Even in a highly critical review of acupuncture in *Nature* magazine in 1980, the authors admitted that "there is no doubt that powerful analgesia with acupuncture does occur and has to be explained."

One explanation is that acupuncture treatment somehow causes levels of beta-endorphin in the body to increase, and that in turn causes a decrease in the pain. British doctors in London and Hong Kong set out to see if that was true.

Vicky Clement-Jones and five colleagues first did a clinical study of twelve male heroin addicts, six of whom were undergoing EAP treatment for withdrawal symptoms. (The other six were also in withdrawal, but they didn't get any EAP.) The researcher took blood and CSF (cerebrospinal fluid) samples from all twelve. They also took blood and CSF samples from another fifty people who weren't addicts. These people functioned as the controls in the study.

Clement-Jones and her group first wanted to determine the

blood and CSF base levels of beta-endorphin and Met-enkephalin in the heroin addicts, and compare them to the controls.
Then they wanted to find how electroacupuncture treatment affected those levels.

They discovered that the addicts had elevated levels of beta-
endorphin in both their blood and their CSF, and that electroacupuncture didn't cause any changes in either CSF or blood
beta-endorphin levels. They stayed high. The situation was different for Met-enkephalin. The addicts had normal levels of the
pentapeptide in their blood and cerebrospinal fluid before EAP
treatment. The levels of Met-enkephalin in the addicts' blood
remained unchanged throughout the study. However, successful
EAP treatment for withdrawal symptoms was associated with a
rise in Met-enkephalin levels in their cerebrospinal fluid. That
was true for all the patients studied.

This was the first study to show definite evidence of a release of
Met-enkephalin in living humans in connection with a form of
acupuncture treatment.

It was not Clement-Jones's only study of the endorphin/acu-
puncture connection, though. In another test, she and her colleagues treated ten patients with EAP. Their ailments ranged
from lower back pain to collapsed vertebrae to cancer. All ten of
them had their pain effectively reduced by the electroacupuncture treatment.

Before the treatments began, the researchers checked the
levels of beta-endorphin and Met-enkephalin in the patients' cerebrospinal fluid. They found these levels to be the same as those
of a group of control subjects who were not in any pain.

The patients received the EAP treatment for about thirty minutes. They all reported relief from the pain after twenty minutes.
Later, when their cerebrospinal fluid was again checked, the researchers found no significant change in the levels of Met-enkephalin. They did find a considerable change in the levels of
beta-endorphin, though: in every case these levels rose from the
pre-acupuncture level. In one patient the level more than
doubled.

Where did the beta-endorphin come from in this second study?
The impermeability of the blood-brain barrier to endorphins
suggested it wasn't the pituitary gland. It seemed most likely to

Clement-Jones that other parts of the brain were producing the peptide.

This finding of a rise in beta-endorphin, but not Met-en-kephalin, contradicts the earlier finding with the heroin addicts. It's a puzzle. At least one study—done in 1977 by three Swedish researchers, including enkephalin co-discoverer Lars Terenius—also suggested that Met-enkephalin levels do not increase during acupuncture.

The contradictory results may mean that more than one mechanism is involved. Some researchers have found, for example, that naloxone reverses the pain relief from low-frequency electroacupuncture stimulation, but not that from high-frequency EAP. The analgesia from the high-frequency stimulation, though, was partly blocked by a chemical that slows the body's creation of another neurotransmitter, serotonin.

So Clement-Jones has suggested there are at least three separate mechanisms involved in acupuncture pain relief: an enkephalinergic system in addicts; an endorphinergic system for low-frequency electroacupuncture; and a serotoninergic system for high-frequency EAP.

Other research seems to support the role of endorphins in acupuncture analgesia:

• In 1976 and 1977 three different studies found naloxone counteracted acupuncture analgesia.

• Huda Akil, C. H. Li and two other researchers in 1978 reported that analgesic electrical stimulation of the brain was accompanied by the appearance of beta-endorphin-like reactions in human cerebrospinal fluid taken from the brain's ventricles.

• At the end of 1980 a group of Italian doctors found an increase of beta-endorphin in six patients after acupuncture was used in connection with chest surgery.

• In 1982, following a study of the acupuncture treatment of people with bronchial asthma, three researchers at the University of Colombo and Colombo General Hospital in Sri Lanka concluded that acupuncture has a placebo effect on bronchial asthma.

A lot of controversy still surrounds acupuncture and the role of endorphins in acupuncture. The evidence for a role, though, continues to mount. No less an expert than Avram Goldstein, one of the discoverers of beta-endorphin and the discoverer of dynorphin, thinks that the endorphin/acupuncture connection is the best-documented and most likely of them all.

Pain and Opiate Receptors

With all the talk about acupuncture, placebos, pain pathways and nociception, we should stop for a minute and remind ourselves of what the whole system depends on. It depends on opiate receptors, those "keyholes" scattered on parts of the body's nerve cells. The neurons have a lot of different receptors for a lot of different chemicals, and each set of receptors can often be divided into a series of subpopulations. So, for example, the adrenergic receptors (into which epinephrine and norepinephrine fit) are divided into alpha- and beta-adrenergic. These in turn are actually two further subpopulations: $alpha_1$ and $_2$, and $beta_1$ and $_2$. There are muscarinic and nicotinic cholinergic receptors for the acetylcholine system; D1 and D2 dopamine receptors; and a whole collection of different GABA-ergic receptors. So, too, the body's neurons carry at least three different types of opiate receptors: mu, delta and kappa. And the mu receptor is actually two— mu_1 and mu_2. One man who has done much to improve our understanding of these receptors and how they work is Gavril W. Pasternak of the Sloan-Kettering Cancer Center and Cornell University Medical College in New York. He has also shown how those receptors may be connected with pain-killers, respiratory depression, and the possibility of creating a new kind of pain-killing drug.

One of the well-known side effects of opiate pain-killers like morphine is the way they depress or slow down patients' breathing rate. It's a side effect that can have fatal consequences.

Pasternak has found that the analgesic effect of morphine, the endorphins and the enkephalins seems to be mediated through the high-affinity mu_1 opiate receptors. Morphine's respiratory effects, however, seem to be mediated by the *low-affinity* mu_2 receptor sites and by the delta receptors.

So the endorphins and enkephalins—the endogenous opioid

peptides—cause analgesia by binding with the high-affinity receptors. But morphine causes both analgesia *and* respiratory depression, with each effect mediated by a *different subclass of opiate receptors*. That, to Pasternak, suggests the possibility of someday creating opioid analgesics based on endorphins which are tailored to plug in *only* to high-affinity sites. We would then have opiate-like pain-killers with all the analgesic potency of compounds like morphine, but without the serious respiratory side effects.

Pasternak's findings also raise the possibility of making chemicals that are designed to *block* the low-affinity mu_2 and delta receptors, and *only* those receptors. That would make it possible for doctors to reverse respiratory depression in anesthetized patients without affecting analgesia.

Dynorphin and Pain

Dynorphin is a real blockbuster of an opioid peptide. In standard tests of opiate potency, dynorphin was 50 times as powerful as camel beta-endorphin, some 190 times as powerful as morphine, and 700 times as potent as Leu-enkephalin. It wasn't long before its discoverer, Avram Goldstein, checked it out for analgesic activity.

Goldstein, Barbara Herman and Frances Leslie injected dynorphin-13 into the brains of rats. (To be specific, the peptide was introduced into either the cerebral aqueduct or the lateral intraventricular space of the rats' brains.) The result: catalepsy (another word for total rigidity of the body, a symptom of some mental illnesses) and profound analgesia. As in the early tests with enkephalins, the onset of analgesia was quicker and the duration shorter with the dynorphin than with comparable doses of morphine.

They also injected the animals with a modified form of dynorphin-11, in which they substituted alanine for glycine in the chain's second position. A similarly modified version of Met-enkephalin, DALA, was much more potent than its natural form.

When Herman, Leslie and Goldstein used this "DALA" form of dynorphin, they found its analgesic power was counteracted by naloxone much more rapidly than was regular dynorphin. Goldstein and Charles Chavkin later found that substituting alanine for glycine in position 2 reduced the opiate potency of dynorphin-13, -11 and -10—an effect just the opposite of that observed in Leu-enkephalin. That in turn suggests that dynorphin does not interact with the same receptor site as the enkephalins. If it did, substituting alanine for glycine would have had the same effect in dynorphin as it does in Leu-enkephalin. Whatever pain connection dynorphin has, it is through receptors that are different from those for Leu-enkephalin.

Further evidence for a dynorphin/pain interaction came in December 1981, when Goldstein, Brian Cox and Lawrence Botticelli published a report noting the presence of dynorphin in several parts of rabbit and rat spinal cord. One of the places dynorphin was found was in the dorsal cord. This, as we recall, is an area likely to be involved in the processing and modulation of incoming sensory information related to pain. This finding fits well with the earlier discovery of dynorphin-13 analgesia made by Goldstein, Herman and Leslie. It's likely that dynorphin is deeply involved in some way in the process by which our bodies modify our perceptions of pain.

Enkephalin and Cats, Endorphin and Camels

Researchers continue to explore the physical process and mechanisms of pain transmission, and how and where opioid peptides are involved. Two people deeply involved in this work are Ellen Glazer and Allan Basbaum of the University of California at San Francisco.

They have discovered an extensive distribution of Leu-enkephalin in the so-called "marginal layers" of cats' spinal cords. Many of these "enkephalin-containing marginal neurons" seem to have extremely long axons. Rather than being just "local circuit" neurons in the spinal cord, they may well extend their enkephalin influence to other levels of the spine, perhaps as far as the brainstem and even into the thalamus.

So a nociceptor, probably using Substance P as a neurotransmitter, excites one of the nociceptors in the marginal layer of the spinal cord. The enkephalin-containing neurons in the same region then reduce the incoming input before the signal continues up through the dorsal horn and into the brain via the spinothalamic or spinoreticular pathways.

Finally, after years of talk and experiments on the endorphin/pain connection, involving a half dozen or more of the opioid peptides, we can't help but ask: which of the endorphins are the most potent pain-killers? Which are the least? And how do they compare with the classic one—morphine?

The latest research seems to rank them this way:

1. Dynorphin
2. Human beta-endorphin
3. [D-Ala^2, D-Leu^5]-enkephalin, or DADLE, a synthetic Leu-enkephalin with the structure Tyr-[D-Ala]-Gly-Phe-[D-Leu]
4. Morphine
5. DALA, the synthetic Met-enkephalin we examined at the beginning of the chapter
6. Met-enkephalin
7. Leu-enkephalin

Human beta-endorphin, ranking below dynorphin, isn't the only known beta-endorphin, of course. There are beta-endorphins for many different species of animals—probably all of them, since endorphin-like compounds have even been found in one-celled creatures. So how does the human version compare in analgesic potency to some others?

Like this:

1. Camel beta-endorphin
2. Horse beta-endorphin
3. Ostrich beta-endorphin
4. Human beta-endorphin
5. Salmon beta-endorphin
6. Turkey beta-endorphin

Camels may be ornery creatures, but they're certainly feeling no pain.

* * *

As with so much in the field of endorphins, there's still a lot to learn about the connections between the endogenous opioid peptides and pain. There's no longer any doubt, though, that an endorphin/pain connection exists. The evidence has piled up over the last eight years and it's pretty conclusive. There's also not too much doubt that there's a connection between acupuncture and the action of some opioid peptides, and to a lesser extent between endorphins and the phenomenon of placebo analgesia. And while it may be a while before we see doctors and midwives using endorphin-based pain-killers in their practice, that time may not be as far off as we think.

7

Endorphins and Drug Abuse

The deputy prosecutor sighs, and leans back in her chair. "The technology's just moving too fast," she tells the reporter. "The law can't keep up with it. And our attempts to keep up, often as not, are too much like trying to kill a fly with a cannon."

"Or the Blob with a hammer?" the reporter interjects.

"Yeah. That too." She smiles faintly. "A little of both. Remember the LSD scares of the mid sixties? No. You're too young. I was a teen at the time, and I remember reading all the scare stories in the papers. People going on killing sprees, jumping out of windows, suffering genetic damage, giving birth to deformed babies. Almost all of the stories were unfounded. But police and politicians got so frightened they outlawed LSD outright. Then it became devilishly difficult to find out what it *really* did or didn't do.

"And, of course, as scientists did find out more about it, how it worked in the brain and therefore how the brain worked, did any of it make the six o'clock news? Hell, no! You guys were only interested in the scare stories and the Hell's Angels and Owsley and Ken Kesey."

"Hey! Wait a second! I wasn't even born then!"

"Well, you know what I mean."

"And now, with the spread of the ability to make large quantities of synthetic endorphin, and especially this viciously addictive one—"

"—EKZ—"

"—right, 'Enkephalin Z,' Congress has passed this new anti-enkephalin law. And you think it's a repeat of the LSD scares of the sixties."

"What? Oh, no. No, you've got me wrong. I think it's just the opposite. I don't think Congress has gone far enough. This is a poorly written law, Mr. McNamara. It bans the sale or use of *enkephalins,* but says nothing about the *other internal opiates.*"

* * *

The connection between the endorphins and drug abuse seems an obvious one. Opiate drugs like morphine must do what they do in the body by interacting with receptors in the cells. Avram Goldstein proposed a way to find those receptors and three separate teams found them. When researchers went looking for the natural "ligands" for the receptors, the body's own internal opiate drugs, they soon found them, too. And these did indeed meet the criteria for opiate-like chemicals. Injected into experimental animals and into humans, the enkephalins and endorphins had effects similar to those of morphine: they reduced pain, induced physical states similar to those seen in some mental illnesses, and perhaps even relieved some of the symptoms of those afflictions. It seemed only natural to assume the endorphins would have something to do with still another aspect of opiate drug use—addiction to and abuse of those substances.

Some Facts and Numbers

Despite recent evidence that drug use by young people is decreasing, abuse of drugs remains a very serious problem in the United States and many other countries. The most current figures from the U.S. National Institute on Drug Abuse are, to pardon a poor-taste pun, depressing:

• Of those who are twelve to seventeen years old, 37 percent use alcohol regularly; 16 percent are current marijuana users; 12

percent are current cigarette smokers; and 2 percent use hallucinogens.

· In the eighteen-to-twenty-five age group, nearly 76 percent are currently using alcohol; 42 percent are current smokers of tobacco and 35 percent smoke cannabis; more than 9 percent are regular cocaine users; and 4 percent currently use hallucinogens. Prescription tranquilizers, stimulants and sedatives are used by 2 to 4 percent.

· Of those in the population who are twenty-six or older, 61 percent are current users of alcohol; 36 percent, of tobacco; and 6 percent, of marijuana.

Alcohol, cigarettes, marijuana and prescription drugs rank at the top of abused drugs in this country, with cocaine coming on fast. It's difficult to know for certain how serious prescription drug abuse is, since it is grossly underreported to appropriate agencies. How many housewives, business people and students are there who are addicted to Valium, Percodan, uppers, "tranks"? No one really knows, but it's certainly in the millions. More than $12 *billion* was spent in 1980 on prescription drugs.

Marijuana? In 1980 there were more than thirty million people in the United States between the ages of eighteen and twenty-four. If the government figures are anywhere near accurate, about 35 percent of them, or better than ten and a half million young men and women, are current marijuana users. The number who are chronic pot smokers must be much smaller; but even 10 percent of that is a million people who find they can't get through a normal day without five or six joints. And that's just marijuana. What about other illegal drugs: heroin, PCP, cocaine? More than half a million people were arrested in 1980 for drug abuse violations; nearly 19,000 were under eighteen. In 1980 more than $510 million was spent by 3,449 drug abuse treatment units to treat almost 182,000 people.

The numbers for alcohol use are equally distressing. More than three quarters of those who are eighteen to twenty-five years old are current alcohol users. That's twenty-three million men and women. They're not all alcoholics, of course. But consider this: according to one survey, of the forty-two million people between twenty and twenty-five years of age who do drink, nearly eighteen million have five or more drinks at one sitting. In 1980 more than a million people were arrested for drunk driving; 23,000 of them were under eighteen.

Cigarette smoking isn't illegal; you can't get arrested for smoking and driving. But tobacco addiction is as real as the addiction to heroin. Fifty-two million people in the United States are cigarette smokers; fifteen million smoke under half a pack a day; seven million smoke a pack and a half or more per day. They may say they're not addicted, that they can quit any time they want; but anyone who smokes more than thirty-five cigarettes a day is as addicted as the man who *has* to have two scotch-and-waters when he gets home from work, and another three after dinner.

A neurochemical connection exists between the actions of opiate drugs and the endorphins. Just what that connection actually is, and how it works, is something now beginning to become clear. The connection is not simple or straightforward, but it is there. We know enough about the actions of some drugs in the brain to make some reasonable-sounding hypotheses as to how they may work.

Definition

According to *Taber's Cyclopedic Medical Dictionary* (p. 32), addiction is "physical or psychological, or both, dependence on a substance, esp. alcohol or drugs, with use of increasing amounts." Drug addiction, says the *McGraw-Hill Encyclopedia of Science and Technology* (vol. 4, p. 395), is "the state wherein a person is unable to live without the drug in question and is compelled to take it." *Taber's* defines drug addiction as "a condition caused by excessive or continued use of habit-forming drugs." Drug abuse in the same volume is defined as "the use or overuse, usually by self-administration, of any drug in a manner that deviates from the prescribed pattern."

Those are some official definitions, and they all speak of excessive involvement with *substances.* Other definitions of addiction are broader. They include within their purview such things as alcoholism, criminal behavior, fascination with electronic media and video games, gambling, meditation and other forms of spirituality, playing Rubik's Cube, risk-taking, running, smoking, and suicide. One particularly intriguing definition comes from Drs. Harvey Milkman and Stanley Sunderwirth in a 1982 article in the *Journal of Psychoactive Drugs*. Milkman and Sunderwirth speak of addiction as excessive motivation toward satiation or arousal as defense mechanisms. For example, excessive motivation toward satiation would include addictive behaviors such as excessive eating, some forms of meditation and the use of depressant drugs like heroin. As a psychological defense mechanism, satiation-addiction is "defense by retreat." Excessive motivation toward arousal might include risk-taking, gambling, crime, and the use of stimulant drugs like cocaine, tobacco, caffeine and amphetamines. This is "defense by attack."

The interesting thing about Milkman's and Sunderwirth's concept is that they include the biochemical dimension. A person may be biologically predisposed to either satiation or arousal behavior patterns. Early childhood attempts to cope with fear or rejection or other facts of infancy set up psychological patterns of behavior for the person's later life. Those behaviors in turn affect the biochemical balances in the brain's neuronal systems. Those altered balances in turn reinforce the behaviors, and the cycle feeds upon itself. Some substance may block the transmission of signals inhibiting "reward" or increasing "punishment"; other substances interfere with transmission of signals which do the opposite. In doing so they prevent the cortex from knowing the organism has received enough stimulus to be satiated. Or they may keep the cortex from knowing that the organism needs more stimulus. Thus they reinforce the pattern of behavior which led to the taking of the drugs. The behavior patterns get so altered and so heavily ingrained in the limbic system that the cortex cannot effectively signal the limbic system to cease. The "will" is overcome.

Not everyone will agree with classifying contemplative meditation as a satiation-oriented addictive behavior. Some might even question calling excessive fascination with Rubik's Cube an addiction. However, the Milkman-Sunderwirth concept does fit well with what we know of the physiological and psychological effects of substance abuse and addiction. The interaction of behavior, environment, genetic predisposition and neurochemistry is incredibly complex, but it is real, and Sunderwirth and Milkman recognize that.

Addictive substances act directly at the level of the neuron and its receptors and neurotransmitters, and they seem to work primarily in the limbic system of the brain. Some drugs, such as amphetamines and cocaine, cause an increase in the action of the catecholamine neurotransmitter norepinephrine (NE). Amphetamines and cocaine do this through one or more different mechanisms—for example, by blocking the "uptake" or disposal of NE that's just been used and is still sitting in the synapse, or by actually causing the neuron to produce more NE. On the other hand, opiate drugs such as morphine, heroin and methadone act by plugging into the opiate receptors. But no matter what the specific mechanism, substances of abuse and addiction interfere with the normal operation of neurons by ultimately interfering with the process of neurotransmission.

Overload

We know that both endorphins and addictive opiate drugs fit into opiate receptors on nerve cells. Endorphins do it because they're part of the system, and they have certain tasks to perform. They are inhibitory neurotransmitters, making it more difficult for the neuron's membrane to become depolarized and fire off an electrical signal. In this way the endorphin system of nerves acts to inhibit other neuronal systems in the brain. The exogenous opiates, the morphines and heroins and methadones, act upon the opiate receptors because they happen to fit them. And they have similar effects: they inhibit the neurons whose receptors they've plugged into. The problem is that they also overload the system with "fake endorphins." And that just messes everything up.

Let's suppose that you're an endorphinergic neuron, one that uses some endorphin (perhaps Met-enkephalin) as a neurotransmitter. I'm another neuron nearby, but I'm part of the adrenergic system; I use norepinephrine (NE) as a neurotransmitter. NE is an excitatory neurotransmitter; Met-enkephalin is inhibitory. When you release some enkephalin into the synaptic gap between you and me (in response to a signal passed on to you from your neighbor up the line), the peptide plugs into one of my opiate receptors. It keeps my membrane from getting depolarized as fast as it ordinarily might, and so I don't fire off a signal down my length. You inhibit me from releasing NE into the synapse connecting me with *my* neighbor down the line, another adrenergic neuron.

But now the human of whose brain we're a part gives himself an injection of heroin. Those opiate alkaloid molecules pass through the bloodstream and up into the brain, where we are. They filter through the blood-brain barrier and reach us. And there are millions of them! Billions! They float around in the fluid surrounding you and me. When you release your Met-enkephalin as a neurotransmitter, you do it in extremely tiny quantities, because that's all that's needed to make our system work. But this dummy is flooding us out. And those heroin molecules have the same effect on my opiate receptors as does your Met-enkephalin. They plug into them and inhibit me. They are phony enkephalins, fake endorphins.

Well, what can I do? Not much except do what I'm told, and I'm being told to calm down, take it easy; no need to get excited, heh-heh. So I don't. And our boss gets oh-so-satiated; drowsy; "blissed-out"; feeling like he's floating just a few inches off the floor and there's no pain, no pain at all.

And you? Well, there's not much you can do under the circumstances except adjust. You don't need to produce much, if any, enkephalin now. In fact your own opiate receptors are telling you that, since they're equally inhibitory. You're being inhibited from inhibiting, but so what? You're not needed now. The place is saturated with fake endorphins.

But now it's wearing off. The chemicals in the area which break down opioid peptides are finally tearing the heroin molecules apart into pieces that no longer interact with receptors. And now the boss has a problem. He's become psychologically attached to the wonderful feeling of bliss and quietude the smack brings. He'd sure like it again. And then there's you and me. You've shut down almost all production of Met-enkephalin; you're barely working, since you didn't have to. By overloading his system with an external opiate, the boss has turned his internal production of opioids way down. And me? Well, the flood of heroin, combined with its disappearance and subsequent lack of almost any inhibitory peptides, has made me hyperactive. I'm super-excitatory now, firing off at the least interaction of NE or other excitatory neurotransmitters with my excitatory receptors. The upshot is that the boss *wants* more smack, and physiologically he *needs* more smack, and if he doesn't *get* more smack soon he's going to go into opiate withdrawal syndrome.

So he shoots up again; and the cycle continues; you and I adapt some more; the system alters some more; the boss gets more addicted; and on and on and on.

That seems to be the way addiction works; we're not entirely certain of the above scenario, but it does seem to make sense, and it does seem to jibe with some experimental observations. Let's not leave the addict at the point of hopeless addiction, though. For if the person involved in substance abuse wants to stop, and can find help in stopping, that person *can* stop. The essential motivation must come from the addict; it's a real case of choosing life instead of death. But once that choice has been made, the medical researchers can give the person a way to beat withdrawal, and a way to beat addiction.

Enkephalin and Clonidine

Withdrawal is one of the telltale signs of drug addiction, and certainly no fun for those undergoing it as they try to kick the habit. Withdrawal is not simply some groundless psychological state. The symptoms, singly or in combination, include restlessness, irritability, cold sweats, chills, uncontrollable shaking, increased heartbeat and blood pressure and a desperate craving for the drug now denied the addict. At least two areas in the brain have been found to be involved in the withdrawal syndrome: the amygdala and the *locus ceruleus*. The amygdala, we recall, is the almond-shaped nerve knot in the limbic system that is part of the brain's emotional center. The locus ceruleus, or LC, is a dark-colored depression in the floor of the fourth brain ventricle. The LC seems to be a part of the brain's "alarm" function: it helps cause attentiveness, arousal, fear, anxiety, and terror.

Both these brain regions have heavy concentrations of receptors for two different neuronal systems: opiate receptors for the opiate system, and the $alpha_2$ receptors of the adrenergic system, which uses epinephrine and NE as neurotransmitters. The LC in particular has extensions of its noradrenergic neurons (the ones that use norepinephrine as a neurotransmitter) reaching into nearly every part of the cortex. The NE connection is important. As far back as 1915 some scientists speculated that adrenalin (the other name for epinephrine) was somehow involved in the opiate withdrawal syndrome. Experiments reported in 1954 showed that high doses of morphine reduced concentrations of a chemical called "sympathin" in cats. "Sympathin" later turned out to be norepinephrine. In 1970, Julius Axelrod and Ulf von Euler shared a Nobel Prize for showing that NE was a brain neurotransmitter. Many (though not all) studies of the adrenergic system in the 1960s and 1970s seemed to show changes in the brain's use and levels of epinephrine and norepinephrine caused by application of opiate chemicals.

Recently scientists have demonstrated that when addicts (human or animal) begin going through the opiate withdrawal syndrome, the NE-using neurons in their locus ceruleus become hyperactive. Considering the physiological and accompanying psychological states the LC helps govern—anxiety, fear, terror—it's not surprising there's such a powerful connection between this hyperactivity and the withdrawal syndrome.

One way to stop withdrawal symptoms is to give the sufferer morphine, which interacts with the mu_1 and mu_2 opiate receptors. Another treatment is with methadone. Like heroin, methadone is a drug produced from morphine. In fact, methadone is even more addictive than heroin; it simply doesn't have some of the narcotic side effects of heroin. It is a bit ironic, though: the withdrawal effects from deprivation of one opiate drug are alleviated by receipt of another opiate drug. There's also another way to relieve the withdrawal syndrome, and that's with a drug called *clonidine.*

Clonidine was first synthesized for possible use as a nasal decongestant—one of those many things we spray in our dozes whed we ca'dt breedh. It turned out to have other uses, most especially as a treatment for high blood pressure under the trade name Catapres®. During the studies which showed how it worked in the brain to lower blood pressure, researchers found clonidine had a confusing effect on the noradrenergic system. It not only seemed to increase the firing of noradrenergic neurons (acting as an "agonist"), but at the same time seemed to decrease other noradrenergic activities. The reason, it turned out, was that it was acting on two different noradrenergic system receptors, alpha$_1$ and alpha$_2$. The two receptors were located on neurons on different sides of the synapses. Though the same neurotransmitters plugged into them, the results were different.

Clonidine inhibits the firing rate of the neurons in the LC which use norepinephrine as their neurotransmitter through its interaction with the alpha$_2$ receptor. These receptors are "presynaptic": they sit on the axon which is releasing NE and regulate the amount of release via a "feedback" process; and they're also found on the cell body and the dendrites, where they regulate the neuron's firing rate.

Now things begin to make sense. The LC neurons become hyperactive during withdrawal, but clonidine causes an inhibition of noradrenergic neurons in the LC via its interaction with the alpha$_2$ receptors. These are the receptors which both govern the release of NE by the neurons and regulate the neurons' firing rate. The result: clonidine brings the neurons back to a state of relative normality. Withdrawal symptoms vanish.

And what about the known ability of morphine to suppress withdrawal symptoms? Well, remember that the opiate receptors also exist in heavy concentrations in the LC, in the same places the adrenergic receptors exist. Like the alpha$_2$ receptors, many of the mu receptors are presynaptic, and they inhibit the firing rate of the neurons in question. That means morphine and other opiates also act to reduce levels of epinephrine and NE in the locus ceruleus. That's how morphine and methadone reduce withdrawal symptoms.

The thing is, we know the alpha$_2$ and other adrenergic receptors are there in the LC to interact with their natural partners, the catecholamine neurotransmitters epinephrine and NE. And the opiate receptors are present in the LC because they're part of the lock-and-key neural system in which the opiate receptors are the lock and endorphins are the key.

Researchers have found the LC, like the amygdala and other regions of the limbic system, to be practically saturated with enkephalin, which fits into the mu receptors. Enkephalin is an inhibitory neurotransmitter, and the reason morphine inhibits the firing rates of NE-using neurons is that it is mimicking the natural effect of enkephalin.

So it seems that norepinephrine-using neurons in the locus ceruleus have several types of receptors on their membranes: in the places where they receive inputs from other NE-using cells—that is, in their postsynaptic regions—they have inhibitory receptors (called "beta-adrenoceptors" because they are beta-adrenergic receptors) and excitatory alpha$_1$ receptors. On their cell bodies they have opiate receptors and alpha$_2$ adrenergic receptors, both inhibitory. At their output or presynaptic regions—the ends of their axons—they again have those two types of inhibitory receptors.

NE cells lying next to each other can inhibit each other by their norepinephrine neurotransmitter chemical interacting through the alpha$_2$ receptors. They "calm each other down" by "talking" to each other. A norepinephrine-using cell can also be calmed down, or inhibited, by the action upon it of other neurons. Epinephrine-using adrenergic neurons can inhibit them through the alpha$_2$ receptors on their cell bodies. Enkephalin-using neurons inhibit the NE cells through the opiate receptors on the NE cell bodies.

When a person who is addicted begins going through withdrawal, and his or her NE-using neurons in the locus ceruleus become hyperactive, the way to reduce or eliminate the withdrawal syndrome is to calm the hyperactive neurons down. Morphine and methadone do this by plugging into the inhibitory opiate receptors on the NE-using neurons. But morphine and methadone are also addictive. So while the withdrawal symptoms may be alleviated, we still have a junkie.

Clonidine is not addictive. It's not an opiate, it's a drug that mimics the actions of the nonaddictive natural chemicals in the brain and body called the catecholamines, epinephrine and norepinephrine (NE). And clonidine eliminates opiate withdrawal symptoms not by acting through the opiate system but by plugging into the inhibitory alpha$_2$ receptors of the adrenergic system.

Thus it turns out that the opiate withdrawal syndrome, one of the side effects of opiate addiction, is connected to two different neurotransmitter/receptor systems in the brain. These two work together to naturally inhibit the neurons of the locus ceruleus— and a good thing, too! It would be intolerable to go through life in a constant state of fear, anxiety, and terror.

Just ask the people who do. We can find them in the mental hospitals.

For the majority of people, the systems work together well. Quietly, invisibly, using quantities of chemicals so tiny they are measured in millionths of a gram, they keep us on an even keel. We go into alert mode when it's necessary. We feel fear when it's important to our long-range well-being. Our locus ceruleus signals terror when the correct stimulus comes through. The rest of the time—peace, or at least levels of anxiety too low to worry about.

But the person abusing opiate drugs is messing up the system. Instead of receiving molecules of enkephalin, the opiate receptors of the LC get huge quantities of heroin, methadone or morphine. The NE-using neurons become more and more inhibited; less and less norepinephrine gets produced. The neurons adjust and use smaller and smaller amounts of NE. And then the addict is deprived of the opiate. No longer are the LC's adrenergic neurons inhibited by massive opiate doses. NE-using neurons become hyperactive. Fear! Terror! Anxiety! Cold sweats and uncontrollable shaking. Withdrawal. Injections of morphine or methadone will eliminate the symptoms by acting through the opiate receptors. But so will clonidine, and without involving any other addictive drugs. Clonidine slows the neurons down and brings the LC back to normal.

Clonidine's effectiveness in suppressing withdrawal symptoms has led to its successful use in some places as part of a detoxification program for people addicted to heroin, methadone and other opiate drugs. So researchers have, it seems, found a chemical which will relieve the symptoms of opiate withdrawal, and perhaps even get an addict clean, without addicting the person to another opiate drug. We can "cure" a malfunction of the endorphin system by using something that isn't an endorphin.

Endorphins and Alcohol

Addiction to and abuse of opiate drugs like heroin, though dealt with widely in movies, books and magazine articles, is actually not very widespread. Less than one half of one percent of the American populace are heroin addicts. That, of course, is no comfort to them, nor to the people they mug or burglarize for money to support their habit. Even more widespread and destructive to society in general, though, is the abuse of alcohol. When nearly 1.5 million people were arrested in 1980 for driving under the influence of alcohol; when statistics show that more than 14 million people have five or more drinks at one sitting; and when private corporations begin setting up alcohol addiction treatment programs for their own employees—then you know you've got a serious problem.

Alcohol has a reputation for being a stimulant. It's not: it's a powerful depressant. Alcohol causes its effects in the brain by suppressing the activity of the neurotransmitter called GABA. GABA is an inhibitory neurotransmitter, and one of the most important in the brain. Thus alcohol inhibits the inhibitor. The so-called stimulating effects of alcohol occur because the first areas affected by the suppression of GABA are the higher centers of the brain governing self-control and judgment, which are inhibitory functions. Slowing the release of GABA in those areas results in an initial "stimulating" effect. As alcohol accumulates in the brain, though, its inhibitory effects reach to the other centers of the brain. More and more areas of the limbic system and brainstem get inhibited. The person begins having an unsteady gait, confused and slurred speech. Unconsciousness may finally set in. The brain can be so overwhelmed by alcohol, in fact, that it can shut down permanently.

A number of researchers have been looking at possible connections between the endorphin system and alcohol abuse. Some interesting though indirect connections have popped up in some experiments. For example, naloxone will reverse alcoholic stupor in humans. Other experiments have shown that ethanol causes changes in what are called cortical evoked responses in humans and monkeys. Cortical evoked responses have to do with electrical signals in the brain in response to certain stimuli. Floyd Bloom and George Siggins, while at the Salk Institute in San

Diego, spurred on by these and other findings, took a look at the effects of direct application of ethanol to certain brain regions. They found that microinjections of ethanol and ethanol by-products generally caused an inhibition of neurons in most brain regions. This is the same effect opiates and endorphins have. Interestingly enough, there was one exception. Alcohol caused a stimulation of the pyramidal neurons in the hippocampus—which is the same thing endorphins and opiate drugs do there. When they followed the ethyl alcohol microinjections with tiny doses of naloxone, the opiate antagonist often suppressed the effects of the alcohol.

This all suggests some kind of connection between the actions of alcohol in the brain and the endorphin system. But Bloom and Siggins and their colleagues pointed out an important difference between the actions of the two compounds. Endorphins and opiate drugs do not directly change the state of the cell's neuron. They cause changes only indirectly, through interaction with opiate receptors on both sides of the synapse—on the presynaptic neuron (the one releasing neurotransmitters into the synaptic gap) and the postsynaptic neuron (the one receiving the neurotransmitters which have crossed the gap). Ethyl alcohol, though, *does* directly affect the cell's membrane potential, as well as affecting different types of neuroreceptors. Thus the connection between endorphins and alcohol effects does exist, but it is extremely complex. Researchers still do not know for sure how alcohol causes its constellation of effects in the abusing person. Research into the endorphin connection will certainly help answer some of their questions.

Endorphins and LSD

Lysergic acid diethylamide, or LSD, is the most famous of the so-called hallucinogens. Scientists prefer to call these chemicals "psychotomimetic drugs," because some of their effects mimic those of psychosis. Acid is just one of several classes of hallucinogens; mescaline and the amphetamines are another; marijuana and hashish a third. LSD's effects include heightened and vivid sensory experiences combined with a suppression of the ability to make objective discriminatory decisions about the experiences. Control of the inrushing flood of sensorial information diminishes. The redness of the wheelbarrow becomes more important than the wheelbarrow itself, or what the wheelbarrow's used for.

It doesn't take much LSD to cause its effects in the brain; about one nanogram (a billionth of a gram) will do the trick. LSD is not physically addictive, but some people become obsessed with the reality-escape that acid can bring. (Acid isn't the cause of, but rather a tool for, their psychological addiction.) Some people react positively to this shift in reality perception. They find it "enlightening," "mystical." Others don't deal with it so well. Their reactions lead to discomfort, fear, terror, strong mood swings and symptoms of paranoia. The person's mental state before taking LSD is very important in this reaction.

There seems to be no connection between the actions of acid and the endorphins in the brain. Scientists are pretty sure that acid does what it does by interfering with the action of the serotoninergic system—the neuronal network in the brain that uses serotonin as a neurotransmitter. This system exists, among other places, in the midline area of the brainstem. Experiments show that LSD suppresses this region's production of serotonin. Another experiment, in 1980, resulted in the creation of a synthetic version of serotonin which was highly hallucinatory in its effects. One theory for the effects of LSD on the human brain is that the drug imitates the action of serotonin. That fools the serotonin-using neurons in the system and causes changes in the production and use of this neurotransmitter. These changes in turn cause a malfunction of the serotoninergic system, with resulting hallucinations and changes in reality perception.

Other Substances of Abuse

Amphetamines and cocaine. Along with mescaline, amphetamines are a form of stimulatory hallucinogens. Their structure is similar to norepinephrine (NE), and they interact with the adrenergic system. We've already seen the interconnection between the opioid and adrenergic systems in some brain regions, particularly the locus ceruleus and amygdala. In their interaction with adrenergic receptors, amphetamines may well cause changes in the opioid system, too, and vice versa. They also affect the appetite receptors in the hypothalamus, with a resulting suppression of appetite. Cocaine, a stimulatory addictive drug derived from the leaves of the South American coca plant, also involves the action of the adrenergic system. So there may be some kind of endorphin connection there, too.

Phencyclidine (PCP). Phencyclidine is not an opiate drug, but one of a group of compounds called "arylcyclohexylamines." It was first developed for use as an anesthetic, but has in recent years become a drug of abuse. Though some classify it as a hallucinogen, it's not. It's more accurately called a "schizophrenimimetic agent," for it does a very good job of inducing in its users many symptoms of that destructive mental illness. At low (about five-milligram) doses it causes physical symptoms which include agitation and excitement, gross incoordination, catalepsy, catatonic rigidity, and blank staring. Psychologically the user may experience changes in body image, a feeling of estrangement and/or drunkenness, drowsiness, apathy, disorganization of thoughts, extreme anxiety and sometimes hostility and violence. That's just a low dose. At higher doses PCP can lead to convulsions, coma and death.

Just how and where PCP (sometimes called "angel dust," though one must wonder what kind of angel is being referred to) wreaks its havoc in the brain is still not known. Some studies indicate PCP causes a rise in serotonin levels in the brain. Other studies suggest it strongly elevates brain levels of the amino acid tyrosine. Tyrosine is a precursor of both dopamine and norepinephrine, so PCP may cause changes in levels of those neurotransmitters in the brain. Several studies suggest this is so. Other experiments show a possible connection between injection of PCP into the brain and a decrease in GABA levels.

However, most of the studies done on PCP's action in the brain have used the whole brain for analysis, rather than trying to find which parts of the brain may be involved. We don't, in fact, know too much about it. Some have suggested PCP interacts with the so-called sigma opiate receptor. But since there's no conclusive evidence such receptors even exist, we have to take that with some caution. There is in any case no published information linking the effects of angel dust in any way with endorphins, enkephalins, dynorphins or any of the known opiate receptor sites.

Marijuana. This substance is practically ubiquitous—it grows just about anywhere, and its use extends back to antiquity. Marijuana and the other cannabinols are one of the three or four general kinds of hallucinogens, but it doesn't have strong hallucinatory effects unless it's used in relatively large quantities. Usually it makes the user relaxed, giggly and generally "mellowed out." Pot's "munchies effect" suggests a possible interaction of the drug's active ingredient THC with the appetite receptors in the brain. That's just a guess, though. How does marijuana do what it does in the brain? A very good question. If you answer it, there are some folks in Stockholm who may well give you a prize. A number of researchers are currently looking into the neurochemical puzzle of marijuana. Among them is Candace Pert, the co-discoverer of the opiate receptors.

Nicotine. Cigarette smoking may be a bad habit for some; for others it's a real addiction. Nicotine, the active drug in tobacco, is a stimulant that gets into the brain through absorption by mucous membranes in the mouth and lungs. The bloodstream also carries it into the hypothalamus and thus to the appetite receptors. Its stimulatory effects suggest a connection with the adrenergic receptors. There's no published evidence of any interaction with endorphins.

Caffeine. If someone started a Coffee-Drinkers Anonymous, this writer would seriously consider joining. "I'm a coffee addict; I admit it" is something many of us can say. Yes; there may well be a caffeine-endorphin connection, but we talk about it elsewhere in this book (Chapter 10).

Meditation and spirituality. Milkman and Sunderwirth have suggested these may be addictive activities for some people. And they may. But perhaps it's better to consider the possible connections of these activities with endorphins at the end of the book, where we get a little "far out."

Are Endorphins Addictive?

Yes. They are. In fact, a neurochemist studying endorphins found that out soon after endorphins were discovered. In the fall of 1976, Dr. Eddie Wei of the School of Public Health, University of California at Berkeley, reported finding that endorphins act as if they are addictive. Wei took groups of laboratory rats and infused their brains for seventy hours with either morphine, Met-enkephalin or beta-endorphin. Four rats got infused with distilled water as the placebo control group. After the nearly three days were up, the rats rested for about fifteen minutes. Then they were given injections of naloxone, which of course counteracts the effects of opiate-like drugs.

Not surprisingly, nearly all the morphine-injected rats went through withdrawal symptoms: chattering teeth, attempts to escape from the large containers they were in, "wet dog" shaking, and so on. The same withdrawal symptoms were also seen in the rats given Met-enkephalin and beta-endorphin, and then naloxone injections to "shut off" their opiate effects. Thus the two opioid peptides appeared to be addictive in the sense that, suddenly deprived of them, the experimental animals went into opiate withdrawal.

Wei, who has spent many years studying opiate addiction and withdrawal, reported a couple of years ago on another experiment related to endorphin addiction. Wei infused the brains of lab rats with either morphine or one of eight different versions of enkephalin. One was the extremely potent Met-enkephalin analogue FK 33-824. Wei used extremely tiny doses: six micrograms of morphine, for example, and seventeen hundredths of a microgram of FK 33-824. Each rat got infused for three days, and then was taken off the opiate/opioid and given an injection of naloxone to block the drugs' action. All eight of the enkephalin analogues had proven opiate ability, with FK 33-824 the most potent of all. Wei discovered that the more potent the enkephalin was as an opiate, the more powerful were its withdrawal symptoms. FK 33-824 was at the top of the heap.

The discovery of a correlation between opiate potency and addictive potency is an important one. It implies that both effects go through the same receptor. Remember, there are several opiate receptors in the brain and body: mu_1 and mu_2 receptors, delta receptors, kappa receptors and sigma receptors. Each works with different endogenous opioids and each can be turned on by different external opiate drugs. Morphine and its related drugs and Met-enkephalin seem to plug into the mu receptors. Beta-endorphin will bind with either mu or delta receptors. Dynorphin is the endogenous opioid for the kappa receptor, which also interacts with benzomorph drugs. There's still no definite evidence that the so-called sigma receptor is different from the kappa receptor; certainly no endogenous opioid for it has been found. There is evidence that the drug PCP, or "angel dust," interacts with some kind of receptor site in the brain. Whether it's a kappa or a sigma is not known.

Things are even more complicated than this. The two mu receptors seem to be involved in different morphine effects. The mu_1 receptor, a "high-affinity" one, seems to be responsible for the analgesic effects of morphine and the endogenous opioids. Other effects of morphine, such as depressed respiration, apparently are controlled through the drug's interaction with the mu_2 "low-affinity" receptor. Leu-enkephalin may bind with the kappa receptors, since the different dynorphins all have a Leu-enkephalin sequence at their beginning. The Leu-enkephalin analogue called DADLE has been used as a probe to find delta opiate receptors, suggesting that Leu-enkephalin can bind with deltas. FK 33-824 binds equally well with both delta and mu receptors. But a version of FK 33-824 with a glycine at position 5 instead of methionine seems to interact almost exclusively with mu receptors.

If addictive ability is tied to opiate analgesic potency, then the only thing that matters is that the opiate bind with the mu_1 receptor. And if that's the case, there would be no reason for FK 33-824 to be any more addictive than ordinary Met-enkephalin, or the FK 33-824 version with Gly^5 instead of Met^5. However, FK 33-824 *is* more addictive than those other enkephalins; in fact, Eddie Wei's experiment shows it's more addictive than morphine. Could this be because of its ability to bind not only with mu_1 but with other receptors as well? Morphine interacts with both mu_1 and mu_2 opiate receptors, FK 33-824 with mu_1 (since it is very powerful in the opiate "twitch" tests), perhaps mu_2 (we're not sure) and delta. Maybe the truth is more complex than a first glance indicates. It could be that the ability to bind with the mu_1

receptor for opiate analgesic action is the prerequisite for addictive action of an opiate or opioid chemical. The compound's ability to also plug into other opiate receptors then increases its addictive potency.

Scientists have been looking for a nonaddictive opiate that's also a powerful pain-killer for a long, long time. They still haven't found it. Our increasing understanding of the interactions between opiate receptors and exogenous and endogenous opiate chemicals will certainly bring us closer to the day when the search for nonaddictive opiate pain-killers ends in success. Meanwhile, non-opiate chemicals like clonidine are being used with great success to achieve cures from opiate drug addiction. But the only truly successful cure for substance abuse and addiction will be a societal one. For the problems of substance abuse and drug addiction are in the end not physiological but social and ethical—indeed, one might even dare say spiritual. Only when we stop fearing ourselves and others, when we stop hating ourselves and others—only then will we realize we don't need the escapist/ aggressive defense of addictive behavior.

8

Endorphins and Mental Illness

They rolled the cart into the elevator and punched for the basement. Jeanne heaved a sigh of relief. "Good grief," she said, "how do you stand it?" Paul shrugged and smiled a resigned smile at his visitor. "It's not pretty, is it? Well, they're sick people, and sick people aren't a lot of fun to be around." He shrugged again. The light flickered past "2." "How do I stand it? They're human beings. They need help. Some of the people like to read—"

"Some of them like to look at dirty pictures."

"Uh-huh. And for some reason I cannot fathom, a lot of the patients here just love *People* magazine. No accounting for taste."

The elevator stopped and the doors opened. The hospital librarian and his guest pushed the cart down the hall to the tiny library. After it was parked in a corner of the office, Paul collapsed into his chair. Jeanne sat on the corner of the desk. "You didn't answer my question," she said. "Really: how *do* you stand dealing with mentally ill people every day?"

Paul leaned over, pulled open a desk drawer and took out a plastic vial filled with pills. "Prescription," he said. "It's all kosher." He tossed it to Jeanne. She read the label and raised her eyebrows.

"It's only been on the market a few months," Paul said. "It's a beta-endorphin-based compound that some of the people in some of these journals—" (he waved his hand at the shelves)

"—claim will soon replace neuroleptics."

Jeanne's eyes widened.

"Right," Paul said. *"There,* but for fortune and this stuff, go I. That's how I deal with them from day to day, Jeanne. These are my brothers and sisters in here."

* * *

Soon after their discovery scientists began to suspect a connection between endorphins and mental illness. Lars Terenius, one of the discoverers of enkephalins, gave injections of naloxone to two people suffering from chronic schizophrenia. Their auditory hallucinations stopped within minutes. The patients hadn't been given exogenous opiate drugs beforehand, so the naloxone was apparently affecting the levels of enkephalins or endorphins in their brains.

In the fall of 1976, two groups of American scientists reported on experiments that gave added weight to the endorphin-schizophrenia connection. Floyd Bloom, David Segal, Nicholas Ling and Roger Guillemin of the Salk Institute in San Diego injected Met-enkephalin and alpha-, beta- or gamma-endorphins into the cerebrospinal fluid of rats. The animals became highly rigid and immobile. Half an hour after the injections the researchers could place a rat across two metal bookends, with one thin edge under the rat's chin and the other at the base of its tail, and make of the animal a tiny "rat bridge." This bizarre stiffness was almost exactly like that of people afflicted with a form of schizophrenia called *catatonia.* Catatonics are almost entirely unresponsive, and they tend to assume *and remain in* a fixed posture.

Two other researchers, Yasuko Jacquet and Neville Marks, at the Rockland Psychiatric Institute in New York, got results similar to those of Bloom and company. They injected albino rats with beta-endorphin, placing the peptide into the animals' periaqueductal gray (PAG). Mental patients who get doses of drugs commonly used to control the symptoms of schizophrenia often experience a loss of pain. The PAG helps control analgesia similar to this pain suppression. Jacquet and Marks found that rats so injected with beta-endorphin also showed powerful cataleptic-like effects. They had "waxy flexibility": the experimenters could take the animals and literally mold them into any desired posture.

The animals would hold that position for an hour or more after the endorphin injections. They would come out of it only if they were suddenly startled—for example, by a camera's flashbulb going off. Jacquet and Marks had to use very large doses of enkephalins and alpha-endorphin to get even weak cataleptic responses from the rats. But four micrograms of beta-endorphin would do the trick. And—a significant point when we're talking about chemicals that are similar to opiates—injecting the rats with naloxone almost completely reversed the catalepsy-like symptoms.

This kind of behavior, so similar to catalepsy, suggested that disturbances in the amounts or distribution of beta-endorphin in certain parts of the brain was in some way connected to the condition known as schizophrenia.

The Tragedy of "Split Mind"

Schizophrenia literally means "split mind." Its main symptoms are a withdrawal from reality and a severe dissociation in thinking and feeling. Schizophrenics think and speak incoherently. The words are right but they don't connect into anything logical or rational. Their thinking processes become blocked or warped. They lose the ability of rapport with other people; they misjudge what might be called "reality processes." As the disease gets worse their emotions begin to "flatten out." They become very ambivalent and contradictory. The disease climaxes in a total disintegration of the individual's personality.

Standard psychiatric literature identifies four subtypes of schizophrenia. "Hebephrenia" is a form of schizophrenia that affects teenagers and young adults. "Dementia simplex" is characterized by a slow and progressive mental deterioration sometimes associated with mental retardation. (And by the way: mental retardation *is not the same thing* as mental illness. The sooner we unlearn that association, the better off will be both groups of people.)

A third form of schizophrenia is "catatonia," usually characterized by a "waxily flexible" immobility of the body. The fourth form is one most of us are indirectly familiar with from novels, television and movies: "paranoid schizophrenia," characterized by bizarre hallucinations and delusions of persecution and danger.

In recent years many mental health professionals have begun looking at schizophrenia as not one disease, but many. Modern science has been trying for decades to find a cause or cure for this tragic condition—and has succeeded only in developing drugs to control the schizophrenic's behavior. Some psychiatrists and psychologists are now beginning to wonder if the reason no single cause or cure has been found is that there's actually a multitude of abnormal mental conditions, all lumped under the one catchall word: schizophrenia.

Whether it is one disease or many, one thing is certain today: there's no cure for schizophrenia, only treatments for its symptoms. Psychosurgery, insulin coma induction and electroconvulsive therapy (ECT) have all been treatments for schizophrenia; only ECT is still used to some extent. The major "treatment modality" (to use the current jargon) for the last thirty years has been the use of neuroleptic drugs such as Thorazine® and haloperidol. These are basically used to keep the patients from hurting themselves or others, and to suppress their more bizarre behavior patterns. After many years of taking neuroleptics, though, schizophrenics begin showing uncontrolled trembling, muscular weakness and then rigidity—the symptoms, in fact, of Parkinson's disease.

Nature, Nurture and Chemicals

The causes of the schizophrenias are as elusive as a cure. Indeed, if the cause or causes were known, a cure (or cures) would be a lot easier. The "nature versus nurture" battle rages fiercely in this field. Certainly there is a genetic connection. Studies have shown that identical twins have a higher likelihood of both having the disease than do fraternal twins. On the other hand, some psychiatrists claim there is evidence that schizophrenia can be traced to problems in the early development of an individual's personality. And several scientists have found distorted communication patterns in families with schizophrenic members.

Biochemists have spent many years looking into the chemistry of mental illness, and have uncovered impressive evidence that the schizophrenic afflictions are at least in part chemically based. In true political fashion, this neither confirms nor denies either the nature or the nurture hypothesis. But since the brain is essentially an electrobiochemical organ, such work has immense importance in finally breaking through to both causes of and cures for schizophrenia.

The prevailing framework for the chemical understanding of schizophrenia has been the "dopamine hypothesis." Dopamine (DA) is both a neurotransmitter and a hormone. As a hormone, it is produced by the adrenal glands and then broken down to produce norepinephrine (also known as adrenalin). The process of producing adrenalin actually begins in the pituitary gland in the brain, which makes ACTH, a chemical that in turn stimulates the adrenal gland to make DA and finally norepinephrine.

Dopamine and norepinephrine (which is formed from it) have also been identified as probable neurotransmitters in the central nervous system. They are believed to be involved in the initiation and control of motor activity. We do know that a deficiency of DA in the brain is associated with Parkinson's disease, which is characterized by muscular tremors, weakness and finally rigidity.

It is in its role as a neurotransmitter that DA may be involved with schizophrenia. The DA hypothesis basically asserts that *excessive activity of dopamine is a cause of schizophrenia.*

Two major lines of evidence support the hypothesis. First: neuroleptic drugs, which reduce the symptoms of schizophrenia, are known to reduce brain dopamine activity. Other drugs which reduce DA activity in the brain may also sometimes reduce schizophrenic symptoms. Second: cocaine and amphetamines are known to increase brain DA activity, and many abusers of these drugs have learned the hard way that cocaine and amphetamines can cause symptoms indistinguishable from acute paranoid schizophrenia.

The problem with the DA theory is that the evidence for it, while persuasive, is not what the scientific community considers strong enough. Research findings are contradictory; some experiments supporting the DA idea have not been replicated; and much of the work has been done with patients who for many years have been treated with neuroleptics, and neuroleptics alter DA receptor activity in the brain in the first place. It's going to be necessary to find schizophrenic patients who have never been on neuroleptics, and do DA research with them, to really confirm the DA hypothesis.

As more scientists have begun accepting the idea that schizophrenia is not one disease but several, each with a possibly different biochemical basis, other chemical theories have been proposed. Some researchers have found higher-than-normal levels of norepinephrine in the spinal fluid and in parts of the brains of some schizophrenic patients. This suggests that NE may be involved in the disease. Others think a chemical called *phenylethylamine,* similar in structure to amphetamines, may be part of the problem.

Other theories suggest interactions in the brain between two different chemicals. The inhibitory neurotransmitter GABA is one of the most widespread in the brain, and some scientists have found evidence that GABA inhibits the activity of dopaminergic neurons. This has led some researchers to suggest that a decrease in GABA-ergic activity causes an increase in dopaminergic activity, and that *this* leads to schizophrenia.

Another theory involves the balance between DA and acetylcholine, another very important neurotransmitter in the central nervous system. Some researchers have come up with evidence suggesting that if the relative levels of acetylcholine and dopamine get out of balance in the brain, schizophrenic behavior will result.

The theorizing and testing continues. Every time a new chemical is found in the brain, it's looked at as a player in the deadly game of schizophrenia. The newest chemicals nominated for that consideration are the endorphins.

Too Much or Too Little?

Researchers trying to determine what role endorphins might play in schizophrenic illnesses face an embarrassing situation—namely, that both an excess *and* a deficiency of endogenous opiates may be involved. One thinks of the astronomers who, in 1978, discovered a star that seemed to be moving in two directions at the same time. The astronomers solved that impossibility rather quickly; biochemists are having a harder time with endorphins and the schizophrenias.

The evidence linking an excess of endorphin activity to schizophrenic behavior seems impressive, and includes the startling experiments by Bloom, Jacquet and Marks back in 1976. Other investigators have found chemical fragments of opioid peptides present in elevated levels in the cerebrospinal fluid of schizophrenics who haven't had neuroleptic drug therapy. When they *were* given medication for their condition, their levels of these opioid fractions dropped.

Several studies show improvement in schizophrenic symptoms when the subjects get injections of naloxone. Some patients experienced a decrease in their hallucinations; others exhibited a drop in unusual thought content. One researcher reported patients showing "a general improvement in psychotic behavior." Since naloxone counteracts the effects of opiates, these effects might result from a canceling out of the effects of an excess of endorphins in the brains of schizophrenics.

The problem with the "excess endorphin theory" is that the evidence, though seemingly impressive at first glance, is actually not on very firm ground. Many of the findings have not been confirmed by other scientists doing the same tests. Perhaps the effects were the result of extremely high doses of naloxone. Or maybe the methods used were not exactly followed in the follow-on experiments. However, one careful clinical study done in 1978 (when the excess endorphin theory was flying high) didn't find any elevated concentrations of Leu-enkephalin or beta-endorphin in the blood plasma of the schizophrenic patients in the test. That's a flat contradiction of claims supporting the excess endorphin theory.

However, another careful test done in 1979 has kept things in a state of ferment. Jack Barchas, Philip Berger, Stanley Watson and

Huda Akil did a series of clinical studies on fourteen male schizophrenic patients from the Palo Alto, California, Veterans Administration Medical Center. The four researchers gave the men carefully controlled intravenous doses of naloxone or a placebo. The test was tight, and double-blind, and the men were afterward tested for their reactions.

The result? The patients experienced a definite decrease in hallucinations, both auditory and visual. The reduction lasted longer than one might expect from naloxone's action in reversing the effects of opiates like heroin. In fact, the shortest decrease of hallucinations lasted a good three hours. This strongly suggests that an excess of endorphins may indeed be worth taking a look at as a possible cause of some schizophrenic symptoms, for naloxone is the well-known antagonist of opiate peptides.

Once again, though, some cautions—from the researchers themselves. Some of the variables were tightly controlled in this test, but some simply couldn't be dealt with. For example, the people tested had to be ones with fairly constant hallucinations, so the researchers could be sure that any decrease could be attributed to the effects of the naloxone. But schizophrenics who are constantly hallucinating are *not* the norm; so at the very start the four scientists were forced to test their theory on "nonstandard" schizophrenics.

The frequent ratings and tests given the patients over the two days of the experiment were also uncontrollable factors. This repeated testing, the frequent interviews and the effects of starting and stopping this rather limited-duration experiment would tend to cause stress and anxiety even in "normal" people. The effects on mentally ill people could easily alter the way the drug naloxone affected them.

The second version of the endorphin/schizophrenia connection asserts the opposite of the first: that it's a *deficiency* of endorphins in parts of the brain that gives rise to symptoms of the schizophrenias. Here, too, some impressive-looking evidence gets trotted out. Some researchers doing animal studies discovered that the antipsychotic drug haloperidol actually increased the enkephalin levels in some brain areas. The experiments showing cataleptic stiffness in beta-endorphin-injected rats have also been used to support the endorphin deficiency theory. The argument is that this behavior is actually more similar to the stiffness of patients under long-term treatment with neuroleptic drugs for the control of schizophrenic symptoms. In other words, the neuroleptic drugs (the theory goes) alleviate the symptoms of schizophrenias by *increasing* the endorphin levels, pushing them up to a more "normal" range.

Then there's the case of FK 33-824. This is the Met-enkephalin analogue which also has powerful pain-killing and addictive properties. When researchers injected eight schizophrenic volunteers with FK 33-824, the drug reduced their psychotic symptoms. (The study was "single-blind": the doctors knew what the patients were getting—the drug or a placebo—but the patients didn't.) Perhaps the eight people had too little enkephalin in their system, and the FK 33-824 brought those levels up to par.

Another clinical study used an endorphin-like peptide, structurally similar to beta-endorphin but with no opiate-like activity, called DTgE. It's beta-lipotropin[62-77] (or, if you wish, beta-endorphin[2-17]). Six volunteer schizophrenic patients got DTgE in a single-blind test, and eight others got doses of the peptide in a double-blind test (double-blind: *no one* knows who's getting what until the test is over). All the patients in both tests reportedly got some relief from their symptoms of schizophrenia. The implication is that a deficiency of this beta-endorphin fragment was involved in the patients' schizophrenia.

Finally, doctors have been claiming for more than 130 years that morphine, heroin and the like sometimes alleviate schizophrenic symptoms. That, too, suggests there's too little of the endogenous opiates in the brain of the sufferers of schizophrenia.

The problem with the endorphin deficiency theory is, however, much the same as in the case of the endorphin excess theory: contradictory evidence and lack of confirmation. For example, none of those 130 years of reports come from well-designed clinical studies that are double-blind. So they really can't be trusted. Also, no one's been able to duplicate some of the results from many studies that support the deficiency theory.

One of the most widely publicized experiments with beta-endorphin and schizophrenic patients was a single-blind one done in New York in 1979 by Dr. Nathan S. Kline and H. E. Lehman. They gave their group of patients a series of fifteen intravenous injections of beta-endorphin. The doses ranged from one and a half to nine milligrams. Seventy-five percent of them reported dramatic decreases in their hallucinations and equally dramatic increases in their ability to perceive and relate to "normal" reality. So exciting were these results that they were reported in newspapers and magazines around the country.

The story doesn't end there, though. First, a single-blind study of the kind Kline and Lehman did is not as well-controlled as a double-blind experiment. Secondly, their study was with only four subjects—not a statistically significant sample; 75 percent of four people is three people. Thirdly, milligram doses of beta-endorphin are *huge* when compared to their actual concentrations in the brain and nervous system. So Kline's and Lehman's results could well have been the result of a beta-endorphin "overload" of the subjects' systems.

In 1980, Dr. Jack Barchas of Stanford University did a more carefully controlled test with beta-endorphin. Neither the patients nor the staff could tell any difference in effects between the beta-endorphin and the inert placebo used as a control; two different psychological behavior scales showed either no difference or a negligible one; and Barchas and his associates freely admitted that a number of subtle variables and other effects could account for any "improvements" shown in the patients that got beta-endorphin.

That seems to kill the endorphin deficiency theory; but it's still too early to rule it out completely. The variables are still not well known, much less controlled, in schizophrenia tests. A beta-endorphin deficiency *could* be part of the problem.

Complexities and Interactions

The simplistic mind-set is something every scientist and researcher has to guard against. A good theory is going to be the simplest explanation for the greatest number of clinical observations. But nature, though in essence simple, is not *simplistic*. There are often subtle complexities woven into the simplicity of the universe. And that may well be the case with the chemistry of schizophrenia and other mental illnesses. The psychotic mind-set may have not one but many causes; it may result from a disruption not of one brain subsystem, but of the interactions of two or more subsystems.

In the case of the naloxone results of Berger, Barchas and their associates, quite possibly it is not naloxone and endorphins alone that are involved in the decrease of the patients' hallucinations. There could well be an interaction between the endorphin systems (affected by the naloxone) and other neuroregulator systems in the brain. The catecholamine system, which uses epinephrine and norepinephrine (adrenalin) as neurotransmitters, is one possibility. The catecholamine and endorphin systems are both found in the same parts of the brain, so it's quite likely they affect each other. And norepinephrine has been implicated in schizophrenia in at least one study.

Even more complex connections may exist. One such may involve DTgE, which does have intriguing effects on schizophrenics, as the clinical test mentioned earlier showed. David DeWeid, who performed the study, suggests that DTgE acts like the standard neuroleptic drug haloperidol. A year after he reported on that experiment other researchers found evidence that DTgE in fact occurred naturally in the pituitary glands of rats. Then scientists at the University of Arizona, along with Nicholas Ling of the Salk Institute, saw some positive effects of DTgE on rats. Finally, less than two years ago, four researchers from the University of Chicago, the Illinois State Psychiatric Institute and the State University of New York at Stony Brook did a brand new clinical trial of DTgE on humans.

The team studied two separate groups of schizophrenic patients. The subjects in the first group got three- to ten-milligram doses of DTgE once a day for twelve days. In the second test, another group got one- to four-milligram doses for two to three weeks. The people in one group were newly admitted to psychiatric facilities, and hadn't gotten any neuroleptic drugs before the studies began. The other group of patients were already hospitalized at a Veterans Administration hospital.

Two of the eight patients in the first group showed marked improvement; four showed minimal to moderate improvement; and two showed no change. In the second group of seven already hospitalized patients, two showed mild but temporary improvement of their symptoms; four showed no change; but one who had not responded to previous drug therapy showed marked improvement.

DTgE is an opioid peptide *without* opiate effects. How can it have such positive effects on mentally ill people, when it's not a chemical with "drug-like" properties? The answer may lie in a subtle interaction with the brain's dopamine (DA) system.

Back to Dopamine?

One way that opiate-type drugs might either cause or suppress psychotic symptoms in mentally ill people is by interfering with dopaminergic neurons. Exogenous opiates do inhibit the release of dopamine in at least one part of the brain. Though not itself opiate-active, DTgE in the brain may interfere with the actions of dopaminergic neurons, perhaps at opiate receptor sites existing on dopamine nerve terminals. There is a lot of persuasive evidence for the so-called "DA excess" theory. DTgE could be the way our brains deal with potential excesses of DA and keep us from literally going crazy. Most of us, anyway.

It's one theory. It may be wrong. It may be too simplistic to deal with the complex simplicities of schizophrenia. And quite likely it's just one schizophrenia that is caused by DA/DTgE interactions. Others may have different causes—chemical, genetic, environmental, communicative. We have a long way to go to understand the root causes of this tragic affliction; longer to find a cure.

Finally, we should note that beta-endorphin and DTgE aren't the only opioid peptides possibly connected with schizophrenia. Avram Goldstein and Barbara Herman have shown that dynorphin-13 injected into the lateral ventricle of rats causes catalepsy in the animals. Maybe dynorphin is somehow involved in the complex of abnormalities and chemical imbalances that give rise to the schizophrenias.

Our increasing understanding of the endorphin, dynorphin and enkephalin systems, and how they interact with dopamine, norepinephrine, acetylcholine, GABA and other neurotransmitters is a great step in the right direction—into the chemical essence of the brain, and the tragedy called schizophrenia.

Endorphins and Manic-Depression

Evidence—some of it admittedly fragmentary—also points to an involvement of endorphins in forms of mental illness besides schizophrenia.

Some researchers have reported that narcotic antagonists might be helpful in depressive illnesses. Lars Terenius and two associates gave six people suffering from depression doses of naloxone for six to twelve days, with no effects on their mood levels. But when the naloxone was discontinued, two of the six people suffered a worsening of their condition. Since naloxone blocks the effects of endorphins, it's possible the withdrawal of the naloxone caused the patients' endorphins to take effect and worsen their depressive condition.

Nathan Kline gave several depressed patients injections of beta-endorphin and reported some temporary improvements. The test was open and thus subject to uncontrolled variables. Other researchers, though, reported that people suffering from depression became manic when given beta-endorphin injections.

Speaking of mania, several researchers report that treatment with naloxone can dramatically control manic symptoms in patients suffering from this form of mental illness. However, other researchers doing the same kinds of clinical tests report no identifiable effect of naloxone on manic patients.

If the positive results are borne out, though, it would make for some intriguing speculation. Manic people treated with naloxone seem to get better; depressed people given naloxone don't, and when the naloxone is stopped they get worse. Is the naloxone blocking the action of endorphins in these people's brains? Is it thus possible that endorphins play a role in the mental illness called manic-depression? Perhaps what is happening is that these people's endorphin levels fluctuate from too much to too little. This could be occurring not throughout the entire brain, but in areas such as the hypothalamus and the amygdala, which are regions of the brain that regulate emotions. The result of the fluctuations: dramatic mood swings.

The standard treatment for manic-depression today is regular ingestion of lithium salts. It seems to level out the mood swings, and manic-depressive people who regularly take their lithium tablets function as normally as anyone else. No one really knows why lithium works to control manic-depression. But four researchers, including J. S. Hong and E. Costa of St. Elizabeth's Hospital in Washington, D.C., have shown that treatment with lithium does cause changes in the levels of Met-enkephalin in certain parts of the brains of experimental rats. So it seems there's some real connection there, and it bears a closer look.

Endorphins and Electroshock

One of the most controversial treatments for schizophrenia and some other mental illnesses has been electroconvulsive therapy, or ECT, the induction of convulsive seizures in a person by passing an electrical current or electroconvulsive shocks (ECS) through the brain. Some people claim that ECT is an effective treatment for schizophrenic symptoms; others charge that the "treatment" is nothing more than a cruel electrical scrambling of the person's mind and memories, and in the end is worse than the disease it purports to treat. The generally negative portrayal of ECT in popular literature and entertainment (for example, the book and movie *One Flew Over the Cuckoo's Nest)* has mainly served to make the popular conceptions of electroconvulsive shock therapy a very negative one.

There *are* data supporting ECT as a helpful mode of treatment for some mental illnesses in some cases. This record of success naturally led some investigators to look for possible connections between ECS and endorphin levels in the brain.

J. S. Hong and E. Costa of St. Elizabeth's Hospital, along with J. C. Gillin and H.-Y. T. Yang of the National Institute of Mental Health in Washington, D.C., took a look at the question by using experimental rats. They found that repeated ECS caused an increase in the levels of Met-enkephalin in certain areas of the rats' brains, particularly in the hypothalamus and parts of the limbic system such as the amygdala. That in itself was an interesting finding; more exciting, though, was the time pattern.

The temporal pattern of the Met-enkephalin increase, the four researchers found, was very much like the time it took for ECT to have positive clinical effects on humans. It takes more than one electrical shock to cause any improvement in a person's depressed state; a series of such shocks need to take place before the patient can get any relief from his or her depressed state. The researchers found that a single shock failed to increase the levels of Met-enkephalin in any part of the rats' brains. After six daily shocks, though, they discovered that the Met-enkephalin levels rose by 60 percent in the hypothalamus. Ten daily ECS treatments caused a 100 percent increase in the hypothalamic Met-enkephalin levels. And the increase persisted for six days following the end of ECS.

The four experimenters also found that electrical shocks that were subconvulsive (did not cause convulsions in the rats) didn't change any Met-enkephalin levels in the brain. Such subconvulsive shocks do not have any helpful effects on human patients, either.

Then, as part of the experiment, they gave some rats a pre-ECS injection of phenobarbital, which acted to prevent seizures when the animals were shocked. They found that by doing this they also blocked any Met-enkephalin increase in the rats' hypothalami. This establishes a clear link between the therapeutic effects of ECT and the enkephalin-increasing effects of ECS.

Of course, the drastic electrical discharges that happen in ECT must cause massive changes in the physical state of all kinds of brain chemicals. So it's hard to say for sure that it's the increase in Met-enkephalin levels that is connected to positive changes in patients given ECT. For example, perhaps it is a change in beta-endorphin levels that's the link. Remember, the hypothalamus has high concentrations of beta-endorphin.

But when Hong, Costa and the others examined the hypothalami of the rats, they found an increase *only in Met-enkephalin levels.* The levels of beta-endorphin were unaffected by ECS. This suggests that ECT is more limited in its effects on brain chemicals than we might at first suppose. It also shows that the enkephalin and endorphin systems in the hypothalamus are separately regulated.

Finally, consider where the Met-enkephalin increases took place: the hypothalamus, the amygdala, the septum, and a brain structure called the *nucleus accumbens*. These are all regions of the brain associated with the generation and regulation of emotions. It's the emotions that are seriously affected by mental illnesses like depression and the schizophrenias. And it is the control of emotions that is often improved with ECT.

This set of experiments by Hong, Costa and company, along with their earlier work showing a connection between Met-enkephalin levels in rat brains and the use of lithium for depression, is serious evidence that Met-enkephalin may play an important role in how our brains regulate our emotions. It is still another link in the growing chain of evidence connecting the endorphins with mental illness.

9

Endorphins and Stress

The place is a madhouse of shouting doctors and dashing technicians, of blood and exposed bone and tubes and machines. The untrained observer stands in a corner, cowering and trying to stay out of the way. Trying not to throw up. It's the emergency room of a major hospital. The kid on the table has two bullets in his stomach, a third in his groin, still another lodged somewhere in his left leg. He's fourteen and a gang member.

His skin is pale, his eyes dilated and without luster. One of the doctors shines a penlight in each one. They contract, but oh-so-slowly. The boy's brain is being starved of oxygen. His pulse is weak and rapid, his breathing is shallow and its rate is increasing. His blood pressure is down to eighty and dropping. The people working on him care little at this point about the bullets. They have another problem, more pressing. The kid is in shock, and in deep. If they can't stop it, *and soon,* the boy won't live to see another hour, much less another day.

They work fast, so fast that the untrained observer finds it difficult to identify all the things they do. Doctors and nurses shout instructions to one another, calling out in clipped words and phrases that include medical jargon and unfamiliar names. The untrained observer will find out later that when the young nurse with the short dark hair who had earlier given him the tour (what was her name? Charla?) snaps out a call for "MK 23 14 7, and I want it five minutes ago," she's asking for something new.

She's asking for a Met-enkephalin-based drug that is revolution-
izing the treatment of traumatic shock.

*   *   *

We live in a stressful society. At home, at work, at school, at
play, we subject ourselves or are subjected to stressful situations
of various kinds. At work it may be an irritating boss; at home, a
shaky marital situation; at school, the rapidly approaching dead-
line for a research paper that hasn't even been started; at play, the
physical stress of running a daily ten kilometers. The medical
world usually defines stress according to the tenets of Hans Selye,
who began developing his biological concepts of stress in 1950.
Selye pointed out that stress per se isn't bad; in fact, our bodies
may even need a moderate amount of stress just to keep running
in a healthy, balanced and fit manner. Too much stress, though,
can throw the system out of kilter. And then we're in trouble. The
forces that cause stress (what Selye called "stressors") are both
physical and psychological. Injury, germs and viruses can put the
body under stress. So can fear, anxiety, emotional crises—even
joy.

The body reacts biochemically to excessive stress as it attempts
to regain its healthy dynamic balance. It may manufacture armies
of white cells to attack and devour the invading germs. To combat
a viral infection the body will release minuscule quantities of
interferon. In psychologically stressful situations, hormones may
be brought into play to remedy the imbalance the body finds
itself in.

Selye described the way the body reacts to stress and called the
reaction the "general adaptation syndrome," or GAS. It goes
through three stages:

1. The "alarm action" occurs when the body recognizes the
stressor. The pituitary gland and adrenal cortex produce hormones essential to the "fight-or-flight" reaction it will need to
deal with the situation. These hormones include ACTH and prolactin. The heart rate increases, the blood sugar level rises, pupils
dilate and digestion slows. These reactions are directly related to
the release of ACTH, which is the precursor chemical for epinephrine (adrenalin).

2. The "resistance" or "adaptive" stage is the body's attempt

to repair the damage which caused its emergency arousal. Hopefully the acute stress symptoms will begin to disappear. If they don't, though, the body will ultimately not be able to keep up its defenses.

3. The "exhaustion" stage is just that: if the body can no longer keep up its attempt to combat the stress symptoms caused by the stressors (whether physical or psychological), then it gets sick. The sickness may be mental (various neuroses or even psychotic disturbances) or physical; several kinds of cardiovascular and kidney diseases, as well as some forms of asthma, are in large part related to the body's inability to deal with stress.

ACTH has long been known to be the primary pituitary hormone released in response to stress. Scientists later found that prolactin and growth hormone are also sometimes released into the body in stressful situations. In 1975 beta-lipotropin, the immediate precursor of beta-endorphin, was discovered in the blood of stressed subjects. Then, in 1977, two groups of researchers—one an eight-person team from the Salk Institute that included Roger Guillemin, Floyd Bloom and Nicholas Ling—announced that the pituitary gland releases beta-endorphin in response to stress at the same time that it releases ACTH. Later evidence showed that the endorphin and ACTH were released in nearly equimolar amounts.

In the last seven years beta-endorphin has been found associated with a wide range of stressful situations, from exercising and long-distance running to respiratory distress and various forms of blood and spinal shock. It has also been found to be associated with stresses that are truly psychological, such as the fear of impending pain.

Endorphins and the Stress of Exercise

People who do a lot of running for exercise, especially long-distance running, often talk of an effect called "runner's high" or "jogger's high." The longer they run, the more tired they get, of course; but at some point the runners will "push through the wall" and "get their second wind." They experience a renewed burst of energy, and feel as if they could keep on running forever. It's a heady feeling, a feeling of enormous strength and freedom, of almost floating a few inches above the ground. It is, in fact, a little like the feeling people get when they're high on heroin or other opiate drugs. It deserves the name "runner's high." The euphoric feeling of runner's high, though, may only be incidental to what the body is really doing, which is dealing with a highly stressful situation.

At least four studies done in 1980 came up with data that suggested a connection between increased levels of beta-endorphin and ACTH in the blood and physical exercise, running and endurance training. In one, Steven R. Gambert and four colleagues at the Medical College of Wisconsin in Milwaukee did a study in which five untrained subjects (four men and one woman), twenty-six to thirty-five years old, ran for twenty minutes on a treadmill. The researchers took blood samples before and after the exercise period. They found evidence of a huge increase in plasma levels of beta-endorphin, up to 440 percent. At least one study in 1981 found a similar running/endorphin connection.

Some of these early studies were not well-controlled. The Gambert study used untrained volunteers, but other studies were done on professional athletes. That's fine for them; but what about the rest of us, whose heaviest exercise probably consists of walking from the living room to the kitchen during a break in the football game?

Dr. Daniel B. Carr of Massachusetts General Hospital in Boston, with seven other researchers, set out to see what effects exercise would have on endorphin levels in normal, nonathletic people who began doing physical conditioning exercises. They studied seven women volunteers, from eighteen to thirty years old. None of them had been involved in any athletic training or "faddish" diets; they did not smoke and they weren't taking any medications. They had regular menstrual cycles and they had normal blood levels of all the standard human hormones. They were just healthy, non-exercising American women.

The clinical study lasted four months. It began with an initial exercise session consisting of an hour's pedaling on a stationary bicycle against a steadily increasing work load. The doctors took blood samples before the session and right after it was over, and then a third blood sample about a half hour after the bicycle pedaling.

Beginning with the second month of the study, the seven women began a physical training program, which included conditioning exercises, the stationary bicycle pedaling and running. The conditioning program ran for an hour a day, six days a week, for two months. At the midpoint of the physical conditioning programs, the volunteers repeated the initial one-hour stationary bicycle exercise test. The researchers again took the blood samples before, during and after the Exercycle session. In all, the scientists did this sampling three times: at the beginning of the two-month conditioning program; at the conditioning program's midpoint; and right after the conditioning program ended.

The eight researchers found that the beta-endorphin levels in the women's plasma (the liquid part of blood) took a giant jump during the exercise sessions, as compared to the levels during a control period when the women just sat on the Exercycle and did nothing for an hour. More than that, their beta-endorphin levels were also affected by their two-month physical conditioning program. They had a 57 percent jump in beta-endorphin and beta-lipotropin plasma levels during the first exercise session, before they began their conditioning training; a whopping 79 percent increase at the second exercise session, right in the middle of the two months of conditioning training; and a 45 percent increase at the final session, right after the end of the conditioning training.

The results, in the opinion of the researchers, not only showed that exercise increases the levels of beta-endorphin in the body, but that physical training *augments the effect*. Now, that fits well with the personal observations of people who run daily or regularly for exercise and conditioning purposes. Yes, it hurts; yes, it is sometimes boring; but yes, the more you do it, *the better you feel afterwards*, and the more frequently you "push through the wall" to runner's high.

Not everyone agrees that there's a causal connection between increases of beta-endorphin in the blood of runners and runner's high. Perhaps the most pointed objection has come from Lorin Hawley and Gail Butterfield of the University of California at Berkeley. They note it's an established fact that the opioid peptides are too large to pass through the blood-brain barrier (BBB) and thus migrate from the bloodstream into the brain. And the brain, they say, is where the ultimate action is when it comes to any supposed "euphoric effect" from beta-endorphin.

They make a good point: the BBB *is* an effective barrier and, as we've seen earlier, an essential one, too. But several researchers have now developed ways to "smuggle" drugs across the BBB and into the brain. The technique has been used to slip a chemical similar to dopamine from the blood into the brain. Perhaps the body itself already knows how to do this in stressful situations. A runner's body is under stress, no doubt about it. Perhaps the endorphins in the blood are able to more easily slip across the BBB into the brain under such conditions, and thus give rise to the euphoria of runner's high.

Another, even more important point is that the euphoric affect called runner's high may only be incidental to what's really happening. And what's really happening is that the body is dealing with a very physically stressful situation: running and exercise.

We are not long-endurance creatures, for the most part. We like to take it easy. We can accomplish extraordinary feats, and do amazing things, with short bursts of energy. The stories of ninety-pound women who heave cars up off their trapped children are not urban folk tales. It really happens. People can and do accomplish such feats of strength. Such accomplishments, though, are decidedly non-normal. And so is long-distance running, and steady, hour-long exercise stints. When we do such things, we create abnormal stress for our bodies. And our bodies react as they always do to such situations: namely, with the general adaptation syndrome and its accompanying initial increase in the levels of ACTH, prolactin and beta-endorphin in the endocrine system. Perhaps pituitary-produced beta-endorphin *is* somehow slipping through the BBB into the brain, and there linking up with opiate receptor sites, and producing runner's high. And all of that merely a sideshow to the main act: the body's attempt to deal with the stress of a ten-kilometer run or thirty minutes on an Exercycle.

Endorphins and the Immune System

Three experiments reported in mid-1982 seemed to suggest that endorphins influence the body's immune system—the system that fights disease, an essential part of the second stage of GAS.

A group of researchers at the Oral Roberts University School of Medicine, led by N. P. Plotnikoff, inoculated laboratory mice with leukemia cells. Then they gave one group of the mice injections of Met-enkephalin; another group, injections of Leu-enkephalin; and a control group, nothing at all. The mice in the control group were all dead of leukemia within two weeks, but the mice who received the Met- and Leu-enkephalin injections lasted four weeks. When the researchers repeated the experiment but then gave the enkephalin-treated mice naloxone, they found the mice lived a little longer than the control group, but not much.

That suggests that enkephalins are somehow involved in the way the body fights cancers like leukemia, and the peptide could someday be of benefit to cancer sufferers. In another experiment, an *in vitro* or "test tube" one, Plotnikoff and his associates discovered that enkephalins increase the disease-fighting responses of T cells taken from cancer patients. T cells are one of the kinds of cells in the body's immune system, and are known to play an important role in the body's battle against tumors.

Another experiment involved the connection between opioid peptides and another immune system cell, the B cell. J. Edwin Blalock and colleagues at the University of Texas Medical Branch in Galveston discovered in an *in vitro* experiment that endorphins and enkephalins slowed down B cell production of antibodies, which are the proteins that actually fight disease-causing bacteria and other invaders of the body. This would seem to be a counterproductive activity on the part of endorphins and enkephalins. What the body needs when it's sick is not fewer antibodies, but more. On the other hand, at some point the production of antibodies does have to be turned off. In a related development, Blalock has found that B cells and T cells seem to be able to *create their own endorphins and enkephalins,* and that these peptides are the same as those made in the brain by the pituitary gland.

Finally, a team of researchers at the Scripps Clinic in La Jolla, California, led by Steven C. Gilman did an experiment to see if alpha- and beta-endorphin and Met-enkephalin influenced the reproductive capability of T cells. They found that Met-en-kephalin and alpha-endorphin had no effects on the cells, but that beta-endorphin increased T cell proliferation. That's another indication that opioid peptides have a positive influence on the immune system's disease-fighting capability, at least via the T cells.

Endorphins and Breathing Stress

It happens to mountain climbers sometimes, and sometimes to fighter pilots. Two men getting the space shuttle ready for one of its first launches died from it. It often affects people suffering from asthma.

"It" is hypoxia, or a lack of oxygen. We depend utterly on that simple atom for life itself, and too little oxygen can cause dizziness, deterioration of reasoning ability, damage to the brain and, finally, death. The men who died while outfitting the shuttle had stepped into a part of the ship that had been purged of all oxygen by flooding the area with nitrogen. The point was to prevent the kind of disastrous fire that killed three Apollo astronauts in 1967. The technicians forgot there was no oxygen in the compartment, walked in without breathing masks—and promptly passed out and died.

The same kind of thing affects mountaineers who climb too high without using breathing apparatus. The number of men and women who have died on high mountains because of judgment errors caused by lack of oxygen is legion. Fighter pilots who suffer a malfunction of their breathing systems can succumb for the same reason.

Tragically, the same condition of hypoxia can affect people suffering from asthma and other diseases with associated breathing difficulties, such as emphysema. It is not uncommon for emphysema sufferers to finally die from the effects of too little oxygen, and the same can happen to asthma sufferers.

Associated with hypoxia is a condition called acidosis. Acidosis is the state of excessive acidity of body fluids, especially the blood. Acidosis can be caused by a number of different things, one of which is too much carbon dioxide in the lungs—which in turn is often a result of too little oxygen, or hypoxia. Both hypoxia and acidosis are side effects common to many different respiratory ailments, including asthma, emphysema and lung cancer. When we can't get enough oxygen into our systems, our bodies are certainly under a great deal of stress. And that might mean increases in the levels of ACTH in the blood—and perhaps also increases in beta-endorphin.

In 1977 researchers found that newborn babies with acidosis had higher than normal levels of beta-endorphin in their blood plasma. In 1981 two scientists, Hisashi Yanagida of the Tokyo Kosei Nenkin Hospital and Guenter Corssen of the Maricopa County General Hospital in Phoenix, Arizona, showed the same is true of adults with respiratory problems. They also found something more. Yanagida and Corssen took twenty volunteers with various kinds of respiratory ailments, ranging from lung cancer to asthma, and tested their blood at different times for a number of different factors, including acidity and beta-endorphin-immunoreactivity (which is one way of measuring the presence of endorphins in the body). The researchers also had a control group of twenty healthy volunteers who underwent the same blood tests.

The results were impressive. The *lower* the patients' blood pH —that is, the more they were suffering from acidosis and hypoxia —the *higher* the levels of beta-endorphin in their blood. And the *higher* the pH levels, the *lower* the beta-endorphin levels. The inverse relationship was just like that of the newborn babies in the 1977 study. However, Corssen and Yanagida did more than just one sample on one day. Several days after the first session, they went back and did it again. This time some of the patients had improved and were not suffering from hypoxia and its associated acidosis. In every case reported, the beta-endorphin levels had dropped as the blood changed from acidic to more neutral levels. One patient, in a three-week period, had a drop in beta-endorphin-immunoreactivity of more than 94 percent; another, in just three days, had a drop of 53 percent.

The conclusion, the two researchers said, is that hypoxia and acidosis are pretty obviously stressful situations for people, and the body reacts by increasing the levels of beta-endorphin circulating in the blood. That those levels drop when the stressful situation eases is further proof of it.

However, what beta-endorphin *actually does,* aside from just being present, is still poorly understood. One good guess is that the endorphins themselves are part of the second stage of GAS; their known ability to reduce pain, lower blood pressure and generally calm motor activity may help to relieve the stress which the body is suffering.

Endorphins and Anxiety

You know what it's like: your palms get sweaty, your heart races, your breathing becomes rapid and shallow. What's happening? Nothing—yet. You're *about* to take the SAT exam. You're *about* to reach the top of Space Mountain in Disneyland, and you know what it's like going down. You're *about* to jump out of the troop carrier and parachute into a Middle East miniwar that has suddenly gotten big. You've been told by the man behind the glass window that you will soon be given a mild electrical shock on the sole of your left foot, and you *know* you're *about* to get it.

It's anxiety—the curse of our times, it sometimes seems. We get anxious about all kinds of things; some of them are pretty understandable (Will I pass the SAT? Will my boy be safe Over There?); some of them are pretty ludicrous (Is my tie straight? Does she really think I'm great in bed?). We get anxious. We fear fear. We fear pleasure. We fear rejection, we fear acceptance. We worry ourselves to a frazzle.

Anxiety, worry, fear. They're psychological stressors and they induce stress in our bodies as surely as a microbe or a bullet in the gut. And our bodies react to psychological stress in the same way they react to other kinds of stress. They release, among other chemicals, endorphins.

• At the Max Planck Institute in West Germany, researchers found that levels of endorphins in the blood of university students went up significantly when the students were about to take an important exam.

• Experimental rats conditioned to expect an electrical foot-shock had an increase in brain endorphins when they were placed in their cages and were *not* shocked. The increase was similar to that in rats that were given foot-shocks.

• People put in the rats' situation have the rats' reaction. In one test, six men and women were told during a ninety-minute experimental session that they would soon receive a painful electrical shock to their foot. They had beforehand been hooked up to a sensor that measured the involuntary flexing of a muscle in their lower leg, a reliable measure of a person's expectation of pain. Later in the session some of the people got an injection of naloxone, some a placebo, and some no injection at all. The people who got the naloxone showed increased sensitivity to the pain of the electrical shock as time increased. They were also increasingly sensitive to the *threat* of electrical shock. Naloxone damps down the effects of endorphins, which in turn damp down the person's sensitivity to pain. So the endorphins were not only released in response to the *actual* pain of electrical foot-shock, but also in *anticipation* of the shock.

The body mobilizes itself in moments of emergency; that's what the GAS is for, what "fight-or-flight" is all about. Higher blood pressure, increased heart and respiration rate, speeded-up metabolism—the body needs to be at peak energy, at hair-trigger efficiency. From a survival point of view, the GAS is essential. When we were a species small in numbers and possessing only limited tools, running fast and hard was a good thing to do. Doing it automatically, without thinking about it, was even better. Turning and fighting with a killer frenzy was also something we needed to be able to do, when conditions required it.

Today, conditions don't require it very often. There are few hungry tigers, maddened mammoths and stampeding bison herds to threaten us. The body's fight-or-flight response is not appropriate to the stresses of the boardroom, the bedroom, the classroom. Our stress response has more and more become a problem rather than a solution. Ulcers, neuroses, headaches, heart attacks, strokes, nervous breakdowns—these are the diseases of the late-twentieth-century "civilized" human. These are diseases caused in large part by stress, and aggravated in large part by our body's response to stress.

The release of endorphins is an important *positive* reaction in

these situations. Endorphins can counteract our over-reactions
to psychological stress. They slow our breathing, reduce our
blood pressure, decrease our sensitivity to pain, lower the level of
motor activity. They are, in a sense, our body's own tranquilizers.

Endorphins and the Stress of Shock

Traumatic shock can be caused by any of a multitude of stressors
—a concussion or skull fracture; a compound fracture of a bone;
heart damage; strangulation; a puncture of the body cavity by a
steering wheel column or a surgeon's knife; three bottles of Vali-
um®; frostbite, burns or heat exhaustion; the list goes on.

In most cases of traumatic shock, the critical factor is a loss of
blood and an accompanying collapse of function of the circulatory system. With the loss of blood comes loss of oxygen to keep
body tissues alive. The brain is most sensitive, and its functions
suffer first. Consciousness often gets shut down quickly. The
body doesn't need it to stay alive. It *does* need the delicate dynamic balance of chemicals and hormones, but traumatic shock
throws that into disarray. The system begins shifting into a biochemical oscillation that, if unchecked, will end in death. Blood
pressure swings up and down. Breathing and heartbeat wander
back and forth. Chemical balances oscillate from excess to deficiency. Finally, the body ceases to be a coordinated ballet of finely
interacting dancers and becomes a jostling mob of individual
soloists. It dies.

There is nothing more stressful to the body than traumatic
shock, and the body battles back with influxes of ACTH and
prolactin and other hormones. Including, it turns out, endorphins.

Two people who have done much to reveal the role of endorphins and endorphin antagonists in shock are John W. Holaday and Alan I. Faden at the Walter Reed Institute of Research in
Bethesda, Maryland. Since 1978 they've published reports about
their work on the role of endorphins and naloxone in shock. They
found that injections of naloxone help reverse the terrible drop

in blood pressure that follows poisoning; that opiate antagonists like naloxone are useful in treating shock caused by severe loss of blood; that naloxone acts to counteract the hypotension, hypothermia and hypoventilation of spinal shock. These and other findings suggest that endorphins are indeed involved in some way in the body's reaction to traumatic shock.

It's the contention of Holaday and Faden that naloxone has a therapeutic effect in shock situations because it helps suppress the release of pituitary endorphins into the CNS. The endorphins, like ACTH and other hormones released in stressful situations, act in shock situations to help the body counteract the stressors that are threatening it. The body fights back through the GAS, the general adaptation syndrome. Breathing speeds up, heart rate increases, blood pressure drops, chemical balances change, blood sugar increases, adrenalin races through the system.

But in the situation of the fourteen-year-old boy with the four bullets in his body, those reactions themselves serve only to increase the stress. The boy isn't going anywhere. It's too late for "fight-or-flight." The GAS is simply increasing the blood loss, the biochemical oscillations.

Holaday, Faden and Mary O'Hara performed a simple yet elegant experiment to show how pituitary-produced endorphins act in the central nervous system to produce their shock effects. The three experimenters surgically removed the pituitaries from a group of experimental rats. Another group, a control group of rats, were sham-operated (the surgery went as far as possible without removing the pituitaries). About two weeks later, the researchers subjected the rats to shock by gradually removing some of their blood. They measured the animals' blood pressure, pulse pressure, heart rate, breathing rate, and mean arterial pressure with micro-sized instruments inserted into the rats' blood vessels.

After the pituitaries were removed from the first group of rats, their mean arterial pressure, heart rate and breathing rate decreased. Chemicals produced by the pituitary were supposed to moderate those functions. Now they were no longer being made. After the researchers subjected all the rats to shock, they gave both groups injections of naloxone. The naloxone produced a significant increase in the pulse pressure and mean arterial pressure of rats that still had their pituitaries. It was preventing beta-endorphin from acting on opiate receptors and depressing those bodily functions. But were those receptors in the brain or some-where else—in the intestines, for example, or the spinal column, or the pancreas?

The answer came from the reaction of the first group of rats, the ones who had had their pituitaries removed. The injections of naloxone *had no effect* on their heart rate, blood pressure or any-thing else. The rats were still producing endorphins outside the central nervous system, as were the ones still possessing pituitar-ies. But the naloxone still didn't increase their blood pressure or other functions. Only in the CNS of the rats was the source of beta-endorphin shut off. Their pituitaries were gone. The ab-sence of any naloxone effects could only be due in this case to a lack of *pituitary* endorphins to plug into *CNS receptors*.

But how could the beta-endorphin penetrate the blood-brain barrier and get to the parts of the brain that control blood pres-sure, heart rate, respiratory rate, and the other functions the experimenters were measuring? It turns out that the BBB is not total. There are places in the brain without it. One such place just happens to lie very near the parts of the medulla oblongata which control cardiovascular activities. Holaday believes that beta-en-dorphin sneaks in, through the back door as it were, from the pituitary to this area near the medulla, and there acts on CNS opiate receptors to damp down the blood pressure during shock and other stress situations. And it is there that the naloxone acts to block the action of endorphin. The naloxone counteracts the well-intentioned effects of beta-endorphin and helps relieve the shock condition—at least in experimental rats.

Naloxone isn't the only chemical that slows the release of beta-endorphin in stressful situations like shock. ACTH is part of a complex system that monitors itself with feedback loops. Too much ACTH released into the body is as bad as not enough. We know that the ACTH released by the pituitary gland travels down to the adrenal glands, where it in turn releases different hor-mones into the blood. Some of these hormones are called glu-cocorticoids; they're made in the adrenal cortex. These chemicals will act through a negative-feedback system to inhibit the release of ACTH if the levels of that chemical get out of hand. It's now known that they also inhibit the stress-induced release of beta-endorphin.

Holaday and Faden have also found that the thyrotropin-releasing hormone, or TRH, has the same effect on conscious rats subjected to shock as naloxone has. In fact, they think TRH may be even better in emergency situations than naloxone; unlike the opiate antagonist, TRH doesn't have any side effects on the body's pain system.

In mid-1982 a group of American and Canadian scientists announced another finding related to the body's reaction to shock. They found that the administration of a synthetic form of CRF (corticotropin releasing factor), the chemical that triggers the release of ACTH, causes a dramatic rise in the blood plasma levels of ACTH and the hormone called alpha-MSH. The effects on the release of ACTH are understandable. But alpha-MSH is produced in a part of the pituitary different from that which releases ACTH. And beta-endorphin comes from the same region as does alpha-MSH. This experiment not only strengthens the theory that beta-endorphin is involved in the shock syndrome; it also adds a new hormone, alpha-MSH, to the list of chemicals the body may use to fight stress.

The body's reaction to stress, be it traumatic shock, running, exercise, disease or anxiety, is a complex one. We continue to learn more about it every day. The more we know about how our bodies react to stress, the more the medical profession will be able to treat its effects—and the better we will be able to keep stress from overwhelming us.

10

Other Endorphin Connections

The doctor cocked his head and looked at his patient. "Your blood pressure's still way too high, Rod," he said. "Tell the truth: are you taking your medication regularly? At all?"

The priest grimaced. "Well . . . no. No, I guess I'm not. Taking it at all.

"I don't like the side effects," he continued. "They're really disturbing. And besides, Jim, I'm only thirty-five. And I'm *busy!* Do you have any idea what my days are like? What my *nights* are like? I just don't have the time to take that stuff."

"You're too lazy to take that stuff."

"No!"

"You just forget."

"Well. Yeah."

"You'll have to remember. You'll *have* to remember, Rod. Your age has nothing to do with it. Just because you're thirty-five doesn't mean you can blithely ignore what hypertension will do to you. It will kill you. I've known people who died of strokes at your age. And they weren't under half the stress you are. And I do know how busy you are."

He paused, and a shrewd look came over his face. Rod saw it; a mischievous grin flickered over his own. "What's that about?" he asked.

"Hmmm. I have this idea," the doctor said. "You don't like the side effects of your medication. And you're claiming you're so busy you forget to take it, anyway. O.K., here's a proposition for you. A friend of mine over at the university is getting ready to do a clinical test on a new drug for high blood pressure. You'd only take it once a day, and you'd take it every day for a year. You would have to keep a diary in connection with this—"

"—I already keep a journal—"

"—Good. Interested?"

"What's the drug?"

"Can't say. The test is double-blind, so you can't know. But if you're interested, I'll give you my friend's name and phone number. You tell him I recommended you talk to him about it."

* * *

Much of the early work on endorphins was aimed at exploring their connection with neurotransmission in the brain and with the body's pain perception system. At the same time it became apparent that endorphins had something to do with mental illness, especially schizophrenia, and with drug addiction. Researchers around the world injected various natural and synthetic endorphins into rats, mice and other creatures in attempts to track down those connections.

These aren't the only areas of interest to scientists studying endorphins, though. Years of experimentation and clinical trials have uncovered many other possible roles for endorphins in the body. It now seems these peptides may be connected—though not necessarily causally—to a large range of conditions and processes, including obesity, the effects of fasting, hypertension, anorexia nervosa, arthritis, thermoregulation, coffee drinking, menstruation, and memory and learning.

Endorphins and Body Weight

In 1950 a group of scientists discovered a fat mouse that is different from other fat mice: it is *genetically* obese. It's fat not just because it eats a lot, but because it has a defective gene in its set of chromosomes that produces a *compulsion* to eat a lot. This mutation creates a whole set of bodily alterations in the hapless rodent besides its excessive eating compulsion: so-called "ob/ob" mice also suffer from increased production of fatty tissue, decreased ability to break down that tissue, reduced development of sexual organs and an excessive amount of insulin in the blood.

In the late 1970s, several research teams found that these genetically fat mice also have elevated levels of beta-endorphin in their pituitary glands. That was thought by some people to be a pretty interesting finding. Also intriguing was what happened when normal rats were given injections of beta-endorphin in their hypothalamus areas, where appetite is controlled. The little creatures started overeating. When genetically normal rats and mice were given injections of naloxone their food intake decreased, and this effect was even more pronounced in the ob/ob mice.

All these results led some researchers to suggest that there was a causal connection between beta-endorphin and obesity: namely, that the overweight condition of the genetically obese mice was caused by abnormal opioid metabolism (which, of course, ultimately was caused by the mutated gene in the ob/ob mice); and that beta-endorphin interacted with opiate receptor sites in the digestive systems of the mice, thus playing a role in the regulation of food intake.

The hypothesis was a good one, since the preliminary data certainly supported it. But would additional experiments produce a picture to fit that frame? In late 1978 five researchers at the Salk Institute (Jean Rossier, Joseph Rogers, Tamotsu Shibasaki, Roger Guillemin and Floyd Bloom) decided to check it out. They examined the levels of beta-endorphin, Leu-enkephalin, and alpha-MSH produced in the hypothalamus and pituitary of both a group of genetically obese mice and a group of non-mutated littermates, from one to six months old. The five researchers knew that the greatest percentage of weight gain in the ob/ob mice happens during their first three months of life; if endorphins were a cause of that, their levels would also have the greatest percentage of increase during that time. Earlier experiments had lumped together data from different age groups, so it was not possible to tell from them whether the causal effect was really there. The Salk team's experiment, by zeroing in on the age factor, would clear that up.

The results were a good example of what a well-designed and carefully controlled experiment can show. First of all, the researchers found that the levels of pituitary beta-endorphin, alpha-MSH and Leu-enkephalin were all higher in the genetically obese mice than in the control group of non-mutated-gene littermates. However, the high levels of beta-endorphin appeared only at four to six months of age, up to *three months after* the greatest increase in obesity in the mice. That makes it extremely unlikely that the increase in beta-endorphin is the immediate cause of the mice's fatness. Rather, it seems the other way around: the rodents' excessive obesity is more likely a cause of the excessive beta-endorphin levels. And, of course, the genetically obese mice do have a number of other things wrong with them which could also be causes of the high beta-endorphin levels.

This can rightly be seen as a lesson for both researchers and interested laypeople: it's fun to jump onto the bandwagon; just be sure it's headed in the right direction.

Before we move on to other things, let us not forget about Leu-enkephalin, the third peptide the Salk researchers measured. Here's the kicker: Leu-enkephalin levels in the pituitaries of the ob/ob mice were almost double the levels in normal mice *in the first month* of the obese mice's lives, and that increase persisted. That increase, moreover, correlated highly with increased obese mice body weight. The Salk researchers would not go so far as to say that there was a causal connection between Leu-enkephalin and obesity; but they did say there were good grounds for further investigation of such a possibility.

Is there a connection between enkephalin and obesity? Are fat mice (or people) fat because they have too much enkephalin in their brains? Or is it the other way around, as the case appears to be with beta-endorphin?

It would be wonderful if there were a clear-cut answer, and even more wonderful if the answer were "Yes, too much enkephalin leads to obesity. Here: take naloxone capsules twice a day and *you too* can lose fifty pounds in a month!"

But that's not the answer. There still is no clear-cut yes or no to the question of an endorphin/enkephalin-obesity connection. Sorry. The best way to lose weight is still to count your calories.

Endorphins and Anorexia

Anorexia nervosa has become the "darling disease" of the 1980s, it seems. Everybody's talking about it, writing about it, doing television specials about it, and/or claiming they were/are anorexic "but winning the battle."

Despite the glitter of "chic-ness," anorexia nervosa is not a fun or pretty condition. It is a terrible affliction that kills as many as 20 percent of the people who get it, and most of the people who get it are preadolescent or adolescent girls. The disease has its roots in the mind, but doesn't seem to be associated with any specific neurosis or psychosis. No one really knows why it occurs —only that, for any of a myriad "reasons," the patient decides she's too fat, and so she proceeds to compulsively starve herself to death. She can be treated, and sometimes successfully, with counseling; but the process is long, and traumatic, and not always successful.

The connection between endorphins and anorexia nervosa is indirect at best. In 1981 three British researchers at the Cambridge University's Department of Medicine, Ray Moore, Ivor Mills and Alison Forster, reported on a clinical study of the effects of intravenously injected naloxone on twelve women with anorexia nervosa. The immediate reason for their study was an earlier study that suggested naloxone might have an anti-lipolytic action—it might counteract the breakdown of fat in the body. The researchers figured that if this were true, then naloxone injections might reduce weight loss in anorexic patients by tending to keep their fatty tissue levels up.

The results of the study indicated that naloxone did indeed tend to reduce anti-lipolytic activity in the anorexic women; they gained significantly more weight in the week that followed the start of the naloxone infusion than in the week before, and in the week before the end of the naloxone infusions than in the following week. There was a greater weight gain during the entire period the patients received naloxone than in a similar period afterwards.

This apparent naloxone effect indirectly suggests an endorphin connection to anorexia, because naloxone is an opiate antagonist. If naloxone tends to increase weight gain by reducing the destruction of fat in the body, then perhaps beta-endorphin tends to *decrease* body weight in anorexics by *increasing* the rate of fat destruction.

Does it? In 1979 three other researchers had found that naloxone did *not* counteract the lipolytic action of pig beta-endorphin in rabbit fat cells, and that other opioid peptides didn't even have the same effect on fat cells that beta-endorphin had. That earlier study, though, was done *in vitro*—in a test tube or petri dish, on isolated tissues. The study by Moore, Mills and Forster was done *in vivo*, on living humans. What happens *in vitro* isn't always what happens *in vivo*. And "in vivo" is in the real world. The researchers think it's possible naloxone causes its effect in anorexics by affecting the control of fat decomposition by nerves of the sympathetic nervous system (SNS). That's the part of the nervous system that's involved in adjusting the actions of the heart, blood vessels—and digestive organs. It's also highly active in states of strong emotional content.

In another study reported in 1982 in the *American Journal of Psychiatry*, researchers at the National Institute of Mental Health demonstrated higher levels of opioid activity in the CSF of patients with anorexia than either in the same people after their weight was restored or in a group of normal people. This is further evidence that higher than normal levels of opioid peptides in the nervous system are somehow connected with anorexia.

Finally, there's the very intriguing report in the February 3, 1983, issue of the prestigious *New England Journal of Medicine*. Three doctors in the Department of Psychiatry of the University of Arizona Health Sciences Center—Alayne Yates, Kevin Leehey and Catherine Shisslak—demonstrated fascinating similarities between compulsive runners and anorexics. In discussing endorphins and stress in the last chapter, we noted the phenomenon of "runner's high," and how it may well be connected to endorphins in runners' bodies. Yates, Leehey and Shisslak note that "obligatory runners" resemble people with anorexia nervosa in having personality characteristics such as inhibition of anger, tolerance of physical discomfort, denial of possibly serious injuries or harm, and a tendency toward depression. Anorexics are often compulsively athletic. Compulsive runners are often obsessed with food and put a strong emphasis on staying thin. Anorexics often report feeling a "high" that eliminates fatigue and the need to eat. Not all runners are like anorexics, of course. The majority are healthy, well-adjusted people who enjoy the exercise (and perhaps the high!). But the similarities between *compulsive* runners and anorexics, including the ones connected with endorphins, certainly exist. Perhaps researchers should explore more deeply the relationship between endorphins and compulsive behavior of many kinds.

Endorphins and Fasting

A fairly good case can be made for linking endorphins to feeding behavior. Some 1980 studies show that opioid peptides stimulate feeding in rats that are already full; that opiate antagonists like naloxone suppress feeding in animals that have already been deprived of food and should be hungry; and that rats that are starved experience an analgesic effect which is in turn reduced by naloxone.

One particularly intriguing experiment was done in 1980 by Steven Gambert of the Medical College of Wisconsin. He had already done a study examining endorphins and "runner's high." Gambert and three colleagues, Thomas L. Garthwaite, Carol H. Ponzer and Thad C. Hagen, put a group of rats on a three-day fast, then killed them and examined their pituitaries and hypothalami for any possible changes in levels of beta-endorphin and ACTH. They reported finding decreases in the concentration of beta-endorphin in the hypothalamus but not in the pituitary, and no decrease of ACTH in either of the two locations. Gambert and his associates concluded that hypothalamic beta-endorphin is modified by acute starvation and that the peptide may be involved in the regulation of food behavior.

Not everyone agreed with the conclusion. Floyd Bloom and Joseph Rogers, who'd been among the researchers doing the experiment on the ob/ob mice we looked at earlier, and three other colleagues suggested that Gambert and company were seeing causal connections where none existed. A correlation among data, they rightly noted, is not the same as a cause-and-effect link.

They also mounted a complex statistical argument against the Gambert results, saying in effect that Gambert's statistical analysis of his results was at best incomplete and at worst seriously flawed.

Gambert answered the statistical criticism with one of his own. He also noted he and his team did not actually claim a *causal* connection between the drop in hypothalamic beta-endorphin levels and three days of starvation for the rats (who were caught in the middle of the whole brouhaha and dead to boot). They had simply said that levels of beta-endorphin in the hypothalami of rats are modified by acute starvation, and that hypothalamic beta-endorphin *may* be involved in "the down-regulation of feeding behavior." In other words: "We reported our results and maybe engaged in a little mild speculation."

The whole exchange, by the way, did not take place in secret, but out in the open, in the pages of the prestigious and widely read journal *Science*. And while it probably raised the blood pressure of those involved, it was a pretty typical example of the way science is done these days—in the open, and sometimes with a bit of shouting.

Endorphins and High Blood Pressure

A more recently reported research effort connected to the endorphins-and-fasting question involved rats with high blood pressure. Just as some mice tend to get a lot fatter than normal mice, so some rats tend to be hypertensive—to have high blood pressure. When hypertensive rats go on a fast (enforced, of course, by the humans running the experiments) they tend to experience a drop in blood pressure greater than that of non-hypertensive rats that are on an identical fast. In scientific parlance, fasting has a "hypotensive" (blood-pressure-lowering) effect on both SH (spontaneously hypertensive) and normal rats, but the hypotensive effect is greater in the SH rats. At least three studies done in 1979 and 1980 suggested a connection between increased opiate activity and fasting. Three other studies done in

1974, 1977 and 1978 showed that in both humans and animals the administration of synthetic opiates or beta-endorphin caused a drop in blood pressure and reduced SNS activity. Since fasting animals suffer a drop in blood pressure, perhaps there was a connection modulated by the endorphins.

Late in 1982, Daniel Einhorn, James B. Young and Lewis Landsberg, associated with the Charles A. Dana Research Institute and the Thorndike Lab of Harvard Medical School, published the results of their work on a possible endorphin/blood pressure/fasting connection. First, the researchers measured the systolic blood pressure of SH rats during unrestricted feeding; then, after five days of fasting, they injected the rats with a long-lasting opiate antagonist called naltrexone. Then they measured the rats' blood pressure again. The animals' blood pressure did indeed fall after they were put on a fasting diet, but it rose after they received the naltrexone injection. A control group of SH rats that got only a saline solution injection showed no significant change in blood pressure after the injection. When the same sequence was performed on rats with normal blood pressure, though, the naltrexone didn't cause any significant rise in blood pressure.

This is indirect evidence that endogenous opiates are involved in the drop in blood pressure of the fasting SH rats, since naltrexone counteracts the effects of endorphins and other opiates, exogenous and endogenous. But this opiate-induced hypotension seems to occur only in rats that are genetically disposed to high blood pressure. This is particularly interesting in light of the mounting evidence that some humans may be genetically predisposed to hypertension.

Endorphins, and Learning and Memory

Every time a new neurotransmitter has been discovered in the brain, somebody suggests it may be a memory molecule, or somehow involved in the learning process. Several researchers will perform a series of experiments and appear to prove that contention. Then someone else will point out the flaws in the experiments, the huge overdoses used; and then a *new* candidate appears, and the process begins all over again.

Endorphins have certainly not been an exception to this merry-go-round. In fact, their obvious (though still somewhat fuzzy) involvement in nociception—pain transmission—and the bizarre behavioral changes in rats and other experimental animals that are given intracranial endorphin injections makes them particularly juicy candidates for this kind of speculation. Sure enough, researchers around the world have done dozens of experiments in the last few years, trying to find if and/or how endorphins are connected to learning and memory.

There are two basic motivations for all creatures, humans included, to learn and remember: aversive motivations and appetitive motivations. An aversive motivation is a negative one: "Don't touch the stove, Billie, or you'll burn your hand." Billie touches the stove; she burns her hand. Billie doesn't touch the stove any more. That's an example of aversive motivation. Billie learns not to touch the stove, she remembers what happens if she does. In the world of lab rats, a favorite aversive motivating technique is the foot-shock. The experimenter teaches the rat to do (or not do) something by giving the little creature an electrical shock at the appropriate time. Eventually (and it doesn't take the rat long) the animal learns to do or not do what the experimenter wants.

Appetitive motivation is positive. "If you go sit on the potty when you have to go, Bruce, I'll give you a cookie." Cookies taste good. Bruce gets toilet trained. The appetite that gets assuaged may not necessarily be digestive. Sex is a good positive motivator for learning, too. So is the appetite for love; or warmth; or shelter. In the case of experiments done on lab animals, it's usually food that is the positive motivating force. The researchers will starve the mice for three or four days, then set them to learning a task. The faster they learn it, the sooner they get to eat.

When an experimenter wants to test the possible effects of endorphins or some other chemical on learning or memory in lab animals, he or she will begin by subjecting the laboratory animals to one of these two motivating conditions. Then the researcher, at some point in the experiment, will inject the animals with the substance in question and see how it affects the animals' learning/memory behavior, as compared to a control group that don't get the injection.

We've known for centuries that opiates affect pain perception. They also affect the pain-motivated learning of tasks and behaviors. Opiates and opiate antagonists also have effects on memory in laboratory animals, including retrograde amnesia. An experiment reported in 1979 seemed to show that injections of naloxone increased the retention of *aversively* learned behavior in laboratory animals. Think about it: naloxone counteracts the effects of opiate drugs and opioid peptides, chemicals which *inhibit* pain perception. Naloxone's apparent ability in this experiment to increase retention of behavior learned through aversive conditioning suggests endorphins have a negative effect on aversively learned tasks. Another experiment showed that injecting the opiate agonist levorphanol into the enkephalin-rich amygdala of rats after they'd been trained to a specific task using aversive motivation (a shock) decreased their memory. The same type of experiment, with naloxone injected instead of levorphanol, showed a strengthening of learning and memory.

Other experiments seem to suggest that the effects of endorphins on learning and memory are the *opposite* of the known effects of exogenous opiates like morphine. Extremely tiny doses of beta-endorphin and both Leu- and Met-enkephalin had *anti*-amnesia effects in rats in some tests where peptides were injected under the skin rather than into the brain. Remember the effectiveness of the blood-brain barrier; extraordinarily minuscule quantities of the endorphins were certainly all that managed to get into the brain from the peripheral sites of injection. Yet there was an obvious effect on memory in rats taught tasks using aversive conditioning.

Other opioid peptides also seem to positively affect aversively motivated learning and memory. In experiments done by David De Weid in 1978 and 1980, injections of Met-enkephalin and alpha-endorphin seemed to increase the retention time of such tasks. The amount used was very small: less than three micrograms when the peptides were peripherally injected, and less than one microgram when injected into the ventricular area of the rats' brains. Curiously, *gamma*-endorphin seemed to have an effect opposite to that of *alpha*-endorphin—it increased the rate of "forgetfulness" of the aversively learned task—even though gamma-endorphin is only one amino acid longer than alpha-endorphin. DTgE, a gamma-endorphin analogue, also seems to share its ability to decrease memory.

Do endorphins have effects in appetitively motivated learning? Back in 1976, a group of researchers that included Andrew V. Schally (the 1977 Nobel Prize in Medicine co-winner) showed that some opioid peptides do. They used a test in which hungry rats had to go through a complex twelve-choice maze in order to get fed. About fifteen minutes before the rats ran the maze, the researchers gave them eighty-microgram injections of two different endorphins, Met-enkephalin and a potent Met-enkephalin analogue called [D-Ala^2]-Met^5-enkephalin-NH$_2$. Both peptides seemed to improve the rats' maze-running performance. Another Met-enkephalin analogue with hardly any opiate properties, [D-Phe]-Met^5-enkephalin, had similar positive effects on the rats. Morphine, though, had the opposite result: the rats' performance deteriorated. And in another test reported in 1981 and done by Floyd Bloom and George Koob of the Salk Institute, alpha-endorphin seemed to improve the performance of appetitively motivated learning in rats. Gamma-endorphin seemed to have the opposite effect, but only to a slight and barely measurable extent. However, some tests similar to Bloom's and Koob's seem to show *both* alpha- and gamma-endorphin having negative effects on learning. And naloxone, instead of counteracting this behavior as we might expect from an opiate antagonist, actually increased it.

Many experiments have been done exploring possible connections between the endorphins and memory and learning. Most of these experiments seem to suggest there is a connection; but what the connection really is, is another story. Some opioid peptides seem to increase memory and learning ability, others seem to extinguish it. And sometimes the same chemical does both in different tests. That endorphins seem to have negative effects in aversively motivated behavior may not be too surprising. Perhaps endorphins reduce pain-motivated learning because they are reducing the pain. But why do the same opioid peptides seem to enhance learning and memory in appetitively motivated tasks? A decrease in pain perception is not the same as an increase in pleasure perception.

Obviously, we're missing something. We haven't really gotten to the essence of the connection yet. Perhaps the opiate receptor sites on the brain cells are in some way the key. We have some ideas about where some memory and learning goes on in the brain; and we have a pretty good idea of the location and distribution of various opiate receptor sites in the brain. But any correlations that may physically exist aren't necessarily the key. For memory and learning are incredibly complex behaviors, number one. And number two, not all opiate receptor sites are activated at once throughout the brain. It's a selective process, and depends on what part of the brain is doing what from instant to instant.

Also, we're not talking about one endogenous peptide, but many. At least seven different ones seem to be involved in the learning/memory process. There are probably more. What are the receptor sites for those last two Met-enkephalin analogues?

Other neurotransmitters are also involved in memory; acetylcholine and its associated cholinergic system almost certainly are. The catecholamine neurochemicals, especially norepinephrine, may also be a part of the memory/learning picture. What kinds of interactions are going on between and among all these neurotransmitters, peptides and non-?

The first steps have indeed been taken toward understanding the chemical nature of memory and learning, and how the neuropeptides are involved in it. But the journey is going to be a very long one, indeed.

Endorphins and Thermoregulation

Thermoregulation is the process by which the body keeps its internal temperature at a constant level, a level consistent with optimum performance on a day-to-day basis. If the body's temperature gets too high or too low, the creature will suffer varying degrees of damage, up to and including death. Hypothermia (a condition of lower than normal body temperature) and hyperthermia (higher than normal temperature) are not just strange-sounding medical terms. Lots of people die from them each year.

The hypothalamus is the body's thermoregulatory center. Inside it are tiny groups of cells that monitor and modulate the body's heat retention and heat loss. Information comes to the thermoregulatory centers via the nervous system from temperature sensors in the skin. The hypothalamus is also the place of origin for the precursor molecules that are broken down in the pituitary into endorphins and enkephalins.

Floyd Bloom and three colleagues (Guillemin, Ling and Segal) in 1976, and C. H. Li and two colleagues (Hoh and Tseng) in 1977, showed that both intravenous and intraventricular injections of beta-endorphin produced hypothermia in laboratory animals. Morphine also causes hypothermia, and does so by making the body's outlying blood vessels dilate and thus lose heat faster. Is that how beta-endorphin causes hypothermia?

Li, together with T. M. Wong and A. Koo of the University of Hong Kong, decided to try and find out. They took male hamsters, anesthetized them, and put them in a special cage that exposed one of their cheek pouches to a microscope that was in turn connected to a television monitor. The hamsters were unconscious and felt no pain. Then the experimenters perfused the hamsters' pouches with a special fluid. At different times they added to the perfusing fluid beta-endorphin; Leu and Met-enkephalin; and morphine. The experimenters watched and photographed the results on the TV monitor.

They discovered that all three of the chemicals caused the tiny blood vessels in the hamsters' cheek pouches to dilate. They knew morphine would do it. They didn't know that beta-endorphin and enkephalin would, too; and certainly didn't know beforehand that beta-endorphin would have the greatest dilating potency. Li, Wong and Koo also found that the dilating effect was "dose-dependent"—the more beta-endorphin or enkephalin was added to the fluid, the greater the blood vessel dilation. They also found that naloxone blocked the effect.

Their results showed that endorphins acted on opiate receptors in the smooth muscles of the tiny arteries to dilate those blood vessels. Both beta-endorphin and the enkephalins are produced in the pituitary gland, but enkephalins are very short-lived peptides. So it's more likely that beta-endorphin, released into the bloodstream from the pituitary, was causing the dilation of the blood vessels and thus directly affecting the hamsters' thermoregulation system.

There are a great many differences between hamsters and people, of course. But our thermoregulation systems are essentially the same. So the 1981 Li/Wong/Koo experiment is a pretty good indication that beta-endorphin does indeed play an important role in the way our body keeps its temperature at the right level.

Endorphins and Coffee

This book would not have been written without the consumption of thousands (well, at least hundreds) of cups of coffee. And I'm not alone in my caffeine dependence. In 1980, Americans consumed some 8.1 pounds of coffee per person. That's a lot of coffee, and a lot of caffeine.

Caffeine is a powerful stimulant of both the central nervous system and the cardiovascular system. It fires up the action of the heart; constricts the size of blood vessels; may relieve vascular headaches by this blood-vessel constriction action, or by decreasing cerebrospinal fluid (CSF) pressure; and is a popular ingredient in many pain-relief medications.

It's not too surprising that someone wanted to see what connection might exist between beta-endorphin and caffeine. Caffeine's a stimulant; endorphins seem to function as relaxants—at least they have powerful analgesic effects in many experiments. How might caffeine, with its effects on the central nervous system and other areas of the body, interact with endorphins?

Michael A. Arnold and four colleagues at Massachusetts General Hospital, including Daniel B. Carr, took a look, and published their results in late 1982. First, they determined the plasma levels of beta-endorphin and prolactin (one of the pituitary-produced hormones released in response to stress) in relaxed adult male rats. Then they gently infused the animals' bloodstream with a caffeine solution. Finally, they measured the levels of beta-endorphin and prolactin in the rats' blood and cerebrospinal fluid, to see if the caffeine caused any changes.

It did. The levels of beta-endorphin in the animals' bloodstream rose promptly following the introduction of caffeine, and the levels stayed up for two to two and a half hours. When the researchers infused the rats with naloxone, they underwent a 40 percent drop in their blood endorphin levels. Naloxone also slowed the rise of beta-endorphin levels in the rats' blood after caffeine infusion. However, levels of beta-endorphin in the rats' CSF were not affected at all by the caffeine. Nor were the prolactin levels in either the blood or the CSF.

In another experiment, the researchers took excised rat pituitary glands, put them in petri dishes and treated them with caffeine. This, however, had no effect on beta-endorphin release from the glands.

So it seems that caffeine causes an increase in the levels of beta-endorphin in the body—at least in the bloodstream. Why? For one thing, it's not merely a stress-related response, even though we know the pituitary does release that peptide in response to stress. Prolactin is also released in response to stress, and there was little or no change in prolactin levels in the rats in response to the caffeine infusion.

We know that caffeine affects the levels of several brain chemicals. It increases the levels of serotonin and norepinephrine, two neurotransmitters. Caffeine also reduces the levels of growth hormone (GH) and thyroid-stimulating hormone (TSH). It seems from Arnold's experiment that caffeine doesn't directly affect the release of beta-endorphin by the pituitary. It's quite possible, though, that it affects the hypothalamus instead. In the hypothalamus are produced the precursors and releasing factors for the hormones and neurochemicals that the pituitary releases. It is perhaps these chemicals—including POMC, the endorphin precursor—that are being affected by caffeine.

What this may have to do with coffee drinkers isn't yet known. Arnold's research team used doses of caffeine on the rats that raised their blood caffeine levels to about fifteen to eighteen micrograms per milliliter. That may not seem like much, but it's the same ratio as is found in humans who drink two to three cups of coffee per day. It does make you wonder just what you're doing to your endorphins when you "fill it to the rim."

Endorphins and Arthritis

More than 5 million people in the United States are afflicted with arthritis and rheumatism. Nearly 2.75 million of them are over sixty-five. Often arthritis is simply a bother, a painful condition that an occasional aspirin takes care of. For some people, though, the disease is a real crippler, and the analgesic and anti-inflammatory qualities of aspirin are nothing but a joke.

The widespread occurrence of arthritis and its not uncommon crippling effects make the discovery of a connection with endorphins more than just a medical curiosity. In 1981, Charles W. Denko of the Fairview General Hospital in Cleveland announced that he'd found evidence of just such a connection. Levels of beta-endorphin in both the blood and joint fluids of people suffering from rheumatoid arthritis, gout and similar diseases were considerably lower than their levels in healthy people. More than that: the endorphin levels were extremely low in those who suffered from the chronic and extremely painful versions of these afflictions.

Finding this correlation is not the same as finding a causal connection, of course. And whether the arthritis causes the lowered beta-endorphin levels or vice versa is still unclear; but knowing that endorphins are involved in the pain modulation, and that injections of opioid peptides can lead to profound pain relief, suggests that Denko has indeed found something more than a mere statistical connection. Denko himself has said that beta-endorphin might some day be used to ease the pain of arthritis sufferers. We've already seen that it's been used as a safe and side-effect-free analgesic for women giving birth. A few years from now, when the genetic engineering companies and pharmaceutical houses have begun producing beta-endorphin in commercial quantities, and the price drops, we may well see Charles Denko's prediction come true. And those who suffer from the crippling and painful effects of arthritis will have, if not a cure, at least a new, effective and truly natural pain-reliever.

Endorphins and Menstruation

As we saw at the beginning of this book, sometimes brain chemicals are also used by the body as hormones, and vice versa; and the endorphins are no exception to the rule. The pituitary, we've also discovered, is the site of origin for a lot of those hormones and brain chemicals. That includes not only the endorphins but also gonadotropins—hormones that stimulate the female sex organs, such as follicle-stimulating hormone (FSH) and luteinizing hormone (LH).

Do the endogenous opioid peptides have any influence on the secretion of these hormones in women, and thus on the menstrual cycle? Some evidence suggests this is a possibility. For example, injections of morphine will stop female rats from ovulating. Women addicted to narcotic pain-killers often have abnormal menstrual cycles.

A few years ago four Canadian researchers reported additional evidence of such an endorphin-menstruation connection. J. Blankstein and three associates at the University of Manitoba did a clinical study of twenty-five women. Ten had normal menstrual cycles; thirteen had either an absence of monthly periods (called amenorrhea) or excessive prolactin levels in the blood (the latter is often associated with the former), or both; and two women seemed to be suffering from a deficiency of gonadotropin-releasing hormone (GRH).

Blankstein and his colleagues gave these twenty-five women intravenous injections of naloxone, the opioid antagonist. They gave thirteen other women similar-sized injections of a saline solution; these women were the control group. They found no change in the gonadotropic hormone levels of the women in the early follicular phase of their menstrual cycles. During the later phases of their cycles, though, the naloxone did seem to cause significant increases of LH (luteinizing hormone) in the women's blood after the naloxone injections. FSH levels also increased, but not by much. These increases happened in the women with both normal and abnormal periods, but not in the women with the GRH deficiency.

The strong implication of these results is that the naloxone counteracted the effects of endogenous opiates in the women. The result—an increase in LH and possibly FSH—implies that endorphins act to inhibit the release of these hormones. Endorphins already have a history of inhibitory action, of course, in the regulation of pain. So Blankstein and his colleagues think the results suggest that the endogenous opioid systems in the CNS may help regulate the secretion of LH in women with normal periods. They also think their results show opioid peptides playing a role in amenorrhea, and perhaps in other menstrual abnormalities.

Endorphins and "Thrills"

There's one more possible endorphin connection we'll look at, and it's one of the most intriguing.

Sometimes we describe an emotionally arousing experience as thrilling. Maybe it's when we hear *that* song, or hear *that* voice. It happens when E.T. says, "Come," and the little boy says, "(sigh) Stay." A *thrill*, says the American Heritage Dictionary of the English Language, is "a quivering or trembling passing through the body as a result of sudden emotion." Typically, a thrill is a slight shudder or chill or tingling at the back of the neck. It's usually very fleeting. Sometimes it gets more intense and spreads over the scalp and face and down the spine (yes, a chill really does run down the spine!). Sometimes there's goose bumps, and tears, and a lump in the throat. *Now* you know what we're talking about. Avram Goldstein does, too. The discoverer of beta-endorphin and dynorphin has become interested in thrills, and in the possibility they may be modulated by endorphins.

In 1977, he and Dr. Ralph Hansteen performed some experiments that showed endorphins were probably not involved in sexual arousal and orgasm—a perfectly reasonable potential connection to explore, by the way, considering the effects opiate drugs have on both. But that got Goldstein to wondering about other highly charged emotional experiences, thrilling experiences. If a way could be found to reliably generate and measure such emotional states, it might be possible to find out if endorphins play a role in them.

For Goldstein, music is a potent stimulus for thrills, and that's true of many people. (Judy Collins's "Song for Duke," for example, sends shivers down this writer's spine; then there's Springsteen's "Born to Run," Miles Davis's "Saeta," Billie Holiday doing "My Man," and almost anything by Bob Seger.) In any case, Goldstein set out to explore in a little more detail the mechanism of thrills. First he did a little survey—of the people working with him at the Hormone Research Laboratory; of the medical students at Stanford University; and of the music students at the university. The survey responses gave him an idea of how many people had ever experienced a thrill, and what it did to them, and in what parts of their anatomy they felt it.

After he had that data in hand, Goldstein did a test on ten volunteers in an attempt to see how injections of naloxone would affect their experience of thrills. The volunteers sat in a quiet, darkened room, listening through headphones to music of their own choice. They used hand signals to tell Goldstein when they were getting thrilled, and how much. Then, between two sessions of listening to the same musical passages, the volunteers got an injection—either naloxone or saline solution. Neither they nor Goldstein knew which until after it was all over—in other words, it was a double-blind experiment.

Goldstein found that three of the ten subjects experienced a significant drop in the intensity of thrills after the naloxone injection, as compared to what they felt after the saline injection. Statistical analysis showed this was not a fluke, especially since the same results were obtained in nineteen separate tests. And three years earlier Goldstein himself had shown that people can't distinguish, on their own, whether they're getting a naloxone or a saline injection. So it seems that something real was happening.

It's Goldstein's contention that a thrill is in fact a spreading electrical activity in some brain area which is connected with the regulation of emotions, which is bilateral (since both sides of the body feel thrills), and which is connected with what's called "autonomic discharge" (that is, shivering and quivering). One obvious possibility is the amygdala, a major center of emotional generation and regulation. And we've already seen how the amygdala may have endorphin connections in mental disorders.

So it's at least possible that endorphins, acting in some way via the amygdala, govern the tingling, shuddering feeling of excitement and emotion you felt when Rhett said, "Marry me, Scarlett"; or when Cris Williamson sang "Song of the Soul"; or when you remembered *that* night.

And what about the neuropharmacological basis of some experiences reported by mystics?

Endorphins may be involved in some *very* interesting things. As Mr. Spock would say: "Fa-a-a-ascinating."

TABLE 10.1
MAJOR BIOTECH COMPANIES

Name/Location	Sales, 1982 (Million $)	R & D Focus
Biotech Research Laboratories/ Rockville, Md.	1	recombinant DNA, hybridoma technologies
Cetus Corp./ Berkeley, Cal.	N/A	interferon, proteins and enzymes for oil production and alcohol fermentation, biologicals, pharmaceuticals, etc.
Genentech, Inc./ San Francisco	21	interferon, foot/mouth disease vaccine, human insulin, growth hormones, other medicinal and industrial chemicals
Genetic Engineering, Inc./Denver, Colo.	500	recombinant DNA research for animal and plant agriculture
Genetics Institute	N/A	"Research & Development"
Genex Corp./ Rockville, Md.	6	interferon, other biologicals
International Plant Research Institute/ San Carlos, Cal.	N/A	photosynthesis, salt- and drought-resistant wheat, other agricultural genetic engineering research

PART III

ENDORPHINS
AND BEYOND

11

The Endorphin Business

"Good afternoon, everyone, this is Jordy Guth reporting live from the Martian Stock Market on Phobos via tachyon beam transmission. On the stock market today Endorphin Pharmaceuticals finished up two and three quarter points, at sixty-three and one eighth; Asteroid Mining and Manufacturing was down three eighths of a point. . . ."

* * *

What? "Endorphin Pharmaceuticals"? This must be science fiction. Well, the Martian part and the tachyon part are fantasy, but the business of endorphins is closer than we may realize. How close is a good question. One product of biotechnology, human insulin produced by genetic engineering techniques, is already on the market. Human growth hormone factor is nearly there as well, and various products for agriculture and animal husbandry are in the works. Several types of interferon can now be made in large quantities through genetic engineering of tiny bacteria.

Though the biotechnology business hasn't leaped from the starting blocks into an all-out sprint, it is on the move. Biotechnology products are moving from the lab to the commercial world because people realized they were in large enough demand to make someone a profit. Whether or not we like the idea of improved health care via the profit motive, it's the way things work in this society. They're likely to stay that way. If endorphins are going to make a similar move, it will be for the same reason. And that's a highly likely possibility. We've looked at more than a dozen possible connections between the endorphins and different physiological states and medical conditions. If only a few of those connections bear up under further experimental scrutiny, someone's going to see there's a lot of potential profit in making endorphins available to the public.

But before we delve into future possibilities, let's take a look at present actualities: the business of biotechnology today.

Struggling to Stand

Biotechnology includes several different biological techniques used to produce commercially available products. In one sense biotech has been around since the first farmer began crossbreeding wheat and corn thousands of years ago. And today there exists a multibillion-dollar business in fermentation and other biochemical techniques to produce human and animal feedstuffs, food additives, drugs and medical products, liquor and wine, and the entire plastics mega-industry.

But when most of us talk about biotechnology we mean the technology of today and the near future: the technology of monoclonal antibodies, identical proteins which recognize only one specific antigen and which can be used to diagnose and cure specific and frequently rare diseases; and recombinant DNA, the process of tinkering with the genetic code of some microscopic creature so it will produce a desired compound in large and pure quantities.

Depending on which report you read, there are from seventy-five to five hundred companies of various sizes involved in the biotech field. Biotechnology, generally speaking, is the application of the biological sciences to commercial products and processes. The term is most frequently applied to the use of genetic engineering techniques for the production of chemicals and biologicals currently made by more standard technologies. Most of these products—things like ethyl alcohol, amino acids, vitamins and antibiotics—are made through organic synthesis and/or fermentation technology. These processes have been around a long time, they work well, they're cost-effective and they make the manufacturers a nice profit. Biotechnology, and in particular genetic engineering, which is the process of tinkering with the DNA code of some (usually microscopic) critter so it makes the desired chemical, will have to successfully compete with these more established technologies.

Thus the biotechnology business is still much like an infant struggling to stand up. Sometimes it makes it and then plops back down on its rump. But it keeps trying; keeps falling; and finally succeeds in staying up on its own two feet. Then it's time to learn to *walk*. Even the most optimistic forecasters of the biotech field admit that a large percentage of the companies now in business will fail within a couple of years. The more pessimistic ones see few profitable results from the recent advances in biotechnology before the 1990s.

Predicasts, Inc., the prestigious market research firm, in 1982 issued a report asserting that biotech would begin generating revenues of more than $6 billion by 1985, and of up to $100 billion or more by 1995. Biotechnology's impact will be felt (the report says) in agriculture, with improved crop yields, greater resistance to disease and a higher ability to fix nitrogen. Recombinant DNA could lead to crops that make their own fertilizer, as it were. The Predicast forecast sees $50 billion in revenues in this area alone by the mid-nineties. Genetic techniques could add nearly that much revenue in animal husbandry. Other areas biotechnology will profitably invade include additives for foods and beverages, crop seeds, feed manufacturing and veterinary medicine.

One indicator of biotech's potential profitability is the volume of sales of equipment and systems for this kind of work. A 1982 survey of that field by Tag Marketing Associates in Erie, Pennsylvania, showed $90 million in sales of such equipment in 1981, and a conservative estimate of $140 million in sales by 1985. That's a 55 percent increase in just four years.

However, things are not quite as upbeat as they may seem at first glance. The bloom is off the rose. Some companies have already folded. Others have had to cut staffs drastically and retrench. Still others (like Cetus) have had their big-daddy backers (such as Standard Oil of California) pull out of joint projects. Patent problems have also cropped up in some instances.

The basic problem for the whole biotech industry is moving from R & D through pilot plants to commercial production. It's not that difficult to raise money for research. Research is sexy and exciting. Company flacks throw out terms like "Genetic Engineering!" "DNA!" "Monoclonal Antibodies!" (did he say *clones?*) "Giant Carrots!" "Super-Steers!" "Interferon!" "Cure for Cancer!!!" Venture capitalists get excited. Big companies get interested. The money pours in. The companies make a public stock offering and Wall Street goes ga-ga. Now Genentech and Cetus and Dnax and Southern Biotech have lots of money. And they have lots of project ideas which get the money. Fine.

Then comes the sifting-out stage. Which of these glamorous-sounding ideas will really be commercially viable? The reality of the marketplace comes crashing in. Most of the projects get dumped. The ones that get the go-ahead will need lots more money and time to get off the ground. Ideas for making commercially viable quantities of bulk commodities like ethyl alcohol and biomass chemicals hit the wall. All the talk of a $20 billion market fades embarrassedly into the woodwork. Monoclonal antibodies look a bit more promising, especially for "diagnostic kits." In fact, one company (Hybritech, in California) has six such kits and expects the worldwide market to reach half a billion dollars by 1985. Other companies find possibilities in genetically engineered vaccines for both human and animal diseases. One such vaccine, against an animal disease called scours, is already marketed by Akzo, a Dutch company.

However, the big target for the biotech companies is the $80 billion drug market. A genetic engineering breakthrough here could be revolutionary and very profitable. It takes time—the usual lag from lab to market is eight to ten years—but DNA technology could shorten it. In fact, Genentech and Eli Lilly took just five years to get their human insulin from the test tube to the marketplace. Along with Cetus and Biogen, Genentech is one of the biggest and richest of the new biotech companies. With four hundred patents pending and research moving forward on more than a dozen projects (interferons, hoof-and-mouth disease vaccine, growth hormones and more), Genentech stands a good chance of making it big.

Others have not been so successful. Southern Biotech of Florida went broke. Dnax had to sell out to Schering-Plough. Many other companies have followed similar paths to oblivion and many more will follow in the next few years. Bernard Wolnak and Associates of Chicago, a management consulting firm which specializes in the biotech field, says the possibilities are much more limited than the articles in *Time* and *Newsweek* suggest. The Wolnak report stresses the bottom line—biotech companies will have to compete in the real world, against other companies with years of experience and proven chemical and fermentation technologies. Only a relative handful of genetically engineered products and processes will make it commercially. Only a few biotech companies will make it, too, and those will most likely be ones that strike deals with the already established giants in the biologicals field.

The new technologies will not revolutionize industry. They will, in some cases, make evolutionary improvements and thus make some new products available, as well as making a few older products available at cheaper prices. In fact, Wolnak sees only one area in which genetic engineering techniques may be profitably employed in the next few years: that's in the production of peptide and protein agents for therapeutic uses—things such as hormones.

Perhaps things such as endorphins.

The Humulin® Story

Before we grab this potential brass ring and breathe a sigh of relief, we should look to the current status of just such a product, one that is already commercially available. It's called Humulin®, and it is genetically engineered human insulin made by Genentech, the "super-biotech" company in San Francisco, for development and marketing by the drug giant Eli Lilly. Genentech scientists six years ago jimmied the genetic code of certain microbes and got them to make something they certainly hadn't made before: insulin, and human insulin at that. Insulin, of course, is a hormone made in the pancreas which is essential for life. It assists in the breakdown of sugar in the body. People whose bodies don't make enough insulin will die. The discovery of insulin in 1922 by Canadians Frederick Banting and J. R. R. McLeod was a medical breakthrough of the highest order, and led to the mass production of animal insulin (chiefly from pigs) for use by human diabetics. Banting and McLeod got the Nobel Prize in Medicine the following year.

The genetic engineering of a microbe to make human insulin was another such breakthrough, Lilly and Genentech figured. Human insulin should be better for human diabetics than pig insulin; it would have fewer bad side effects during long-term use because it would have fewer impurities; and it would be cheaper and easier to produce than the animal version. Genentech produced a molecule-for-molecule copy of natural human insulin, then turned it over to Lilly for development and marketing. Genentech in turn was to get about 15 percent of the new drug's sales in royalties.

Humulin® got FDA approval and went on the market in 1982. It hasn't, however, quite lived up to its advance billing. It didn't do much better in clinical trials than the standard porcine insulin. It ran the risk of having its own share of impurities. Eli Lilly allegedly ran into production problems with resulting bottlenecks. And to top it off, by the time Humulin® became available commercially (at a premium price) other companies had come up with new and cheaper ways of genetically engineering human insulin.

Will Humulin® be a commercial flop? It's possible. But even if it is, it nevertheless will have proved something important:

1. Biotechnology can move from the lab to the marketplace, jumping all the regulatory hurdles, and do it relatively quickly. Five years from lab to market is some kind of new record in the pharmaceutical business.

2. Biotech-produced products, and their manufacturers, will have to face and beat the same kind of competition that everyone and everything else does in what passes today for "a free marketplace."

Getting Endorphins to Market

But how do companies go about making commercial quantities of genetically engineered drugs and hormones? It's one thing to laboriously grind up half a million pig pituitaries in order to produce a few micrograms of somatostatin, or dynorphin, or enkephalin. But how do we go from that to millions of ounces of genetically engineered human insulin? Or endorphin-based pain-killers? Or treatments for drug addiction which use still undiscovered opioid peptides?

Genetic engineering, and thus the main thrust of biotechnology, depend on someone figuring out which section of a DNA molecule codes for the particular enzyme, vitamin, amino acid, peptide, protein or other product we wish to make in bulk. In its "host" cell the gene produces only enough of the chemical to suit its own and its body's needs. So when we finally identify that gene we remove it from its normal cell and place it in another one, a cell more adaptable for use in commercial production. Yeast cells are a common host. So are *E. coli*, a bacterium normally found in the intestine and used for years in laboratories in multitudinous mutated varieties. As the cells multiply so do the transplanted genes, and we can speak of these DNA fragments as being cloned. The cells with the cloned genes then produce in large quantities the biological product we want.

The idea is simple. Getting it to work is not. Scaling up from laboratory experiments to industrial production is difficult and tricky. The organisms that normally make vitamin E or vasopressin or dynorphin-A are used to working in the hurly-burly world of the living creature. Multi-liter stainless steel vessels are alien environments. Temperature, pressure and other parameters have to be carefully controlled, or the genetically engineered microorganisms will not produce their product properly—or even at all. And a microorganism whose genetic code has been fooled with so it makes (relatively speaking) huge quantities of interferon is "sick." When 30 or 40 percent of its total output is just one compound, it has difficulty making the other chemicals needed for its own survival. Then there are the problems associated with scaling up from liter-sized flasks, through pilot plants producing several dozen liters of product, to industrial plants with giant vats. Standard mixing technology in industrial fermenters, with impeller vanes stirring the growth medium, can cause damage to the little creatures. Besides, it's not always an efficient mixing method; and it has the problems of waste heat which can kill the microorganism making our synthetic beta-endorphin.

There are ways around these problems, though, and biotech companies are using them. Batch processing is one way of avoiding heat pollution and inefficient mixing. So are processes that use compressed air to mix the growth medium. Other companies are trying continuous-flow production systems. All the while, the companies must make sure they're properly monitoring the process to catch any contamination which can prematurely stop it.

Once the genetically engineered growth medium is properly growing in the industrial vats and producing the desired product, the next step is to recover and purify the stuff. Some cells excrete the product right into the medium. That makes recovery and purification relatively easy and standard. Other cells, though, do not excrete the product of their cloned genes. They must be broken open, and the compound removed. There are hundreds of enzymes, amino acids and other chemicals in the cell from which the desired product must be separated. Purification of proteins in the lab is hard enough. It's extremely difficult in the factory. It is done, of course. Insulin has been purified from pig and cattle pancreases in the factory for decades. But up to now there's been no other source of insulin, so the cost of that process wasn't a factor. If recombinant DNA technology is going to compete, it will have to come up with cheaper and more effective ways of purifying proteins in the industrial setting.

One possible method is by *chromatographic product separation*. In this process the material to be purified is dissolved in a liquid, and the liquid then passes over a series of solid beads of different materials contained in a glass or steel column. Different compounds in the liquid interact with the different solid beads in different ways. Some go straight through without being stopped. Other compounds get slowed down as they interact with various beads. At the end of the column the liquid is collected in different tubes. Each tube will contain a part of the liquid with a slightly different concentration of its various components. Then the process starts over again, with each tube being filtered. Eventually we end up with an almost pure concentrate.

Another method of protein purification which may some day be used to produce commercially available endorphins is *electrophoresis*. This process is based on the fact that different proteins and peptides can be separated from each other by electrical charge. When a mixture of different compounds is subjected to an electrical field, different-sized and -charged proteins will migrate to different electrodes at different rates of speed. There they can be collected in relatively pure form.

Electrophoresis is of only limited usefulness right now, though, because the different streams of electrically charged proteins tend to get smeared together and become less pure. The reason? Gravity. That's why the space program may well come to the rescue of this process and make it the first "orbital industry." Electrophoresis experiments run by Johnson & Johnson have flown on the space shuttle and have been astounding successes. In a sense, it seems fitting that the success of endorphins in industry may well be tied to the success of industry in orbit.

Cloning Beta-Endorphin

The initial step in genetic engineering is to clone the specific piece of DNA, the gene, which makes the product we want to sell commercially. Then the piece of cloned DNA, now removed from the parent cell, must be successfully inserted into a different cell, one which can more easily be used in industrial processes. Scientists first performed this two-stage process with an endorphin-related chemical in 1979, when Nakanishi and his colleagues successfully sequenced POMC, the endorphin precursor.

After determining which segment of cattle DNA held the code for ACTH and beta-lipotropin, Nakanishi and his associates made synthetic copies of that segment and inserted them into a *plasmid*, which they then inserted into the ubiquitous bacterium *E. coli*. A plasmid is a loop of genetic material, a circular piece of DNA carried inside bacteria. The now changed *E. coli* cells produced large amounts of POMC, which the experimenters collected. After performing a complex series of experiments using genetic "probes," they finally were able to read the complete amino acid sequence of the large amounts of POMC which the altered *E. coli* produced.

The use of recombinant DNA techniques made it possible for Nakanishi to make enough POMC for his purposes. But POMC is a huge protein, and beta-endorphin is just a small part of it. For both experimental and industrial purposes it would be necessary to clone the specific DNA segment for beta-endorphin and transfer *it* to *E. coli.* In 1980 a team of researchers from the University of California at San Francisco led by John D. Baxter did just that. It was only the second time that anyone had produced a genetically engineered substance which was active. Gene-spliced insulin, growth hormone and somatostatin had been made before then, but none of it had yet proved to be biologically active. First they used a naturally derived gene for the peptide, from mouse DNA, rather than a synthesized one as Nakanishi had done. The other gene-spliced proteins had used synthetic DNA fragments, not naturally derived genes. Then Baxter and his colleagues spliced the DNA segment containing the beta-endorphin codes into a plasmid which itself contained the code for a bacterial enzyme called beta-galactosidase.

The researchers knew that since this was a mammal gene (mice are tiny, but they are mammals) the bacterium would normally refuse to have anything to do with it. But by fusing the mouse DNA sequence to a bacterial DNA sequence for a bacterial enzyme, they hoped to "fool" the *E. coli* into making a normal enzyme-plus-beta-endorphin. Finally, the researchers attached a "stop sign" to the end of the mouse DNA fragment—what genetic researchers called a "termination codon." This is a common sequence of three nucleic acids used inside DNA codes to signal the end of a particular amino acid production sequence.

The whole thing worked perfectly. The plasmids inside the *E. coli* bacteria happily churned out a protein which had beta-galactosidase connected to beta-endorphin. The team then used a fairly simple technique to split the two compounds apart and *voilà!*—pure mouse beta-endorphin produced by genetic engineering. The researchers then took their beta-endorphin and showed it to be as biologically active as the endorphin produced in the more natural manner inside mouse pituitaries. They had the real thing.

Baxter's achievement points the way to future production of beta-endorphin and other opioid peptides in large quantities for both experimental and therapeutic uses. Endorphin has always been a bit difficult to get, since living creatures make it in such minuscule quantities. But by taking the genetic code for beta-endorphin from one creature and splicing it into another creature such as *E. coli,* beta-endorphin can be biologically manufactured in much larger quantities. And it's just as easy to gene-splice human beta-endorphin genes as it is mouse genes.

Another successful gene-splicing experiment announced in 1982 points to another possibility, custom-made endorphins. Dr. John H. Richards of California Institute of Technology in Pasadena made his own mutated gene, and got it to produce a customized enzyme. He and his colleagues started with the DNA sequence for an enzyme called beta-lactamase. The amino acid in position 70 of this compound is normally serine, and it's followed in position 71 by threonine. In the DNA code for the enzyme, the particular "codon," or nucleic acid triplet, used for serine[70] is "-AGC-," or "adenine-guanine-cytosine." The codon used for threonine[71] is "-ACT-," or "adenine-cytosine-thymine." Richards deliberately changed things. He took out the -AGC- serine codon and replaced it with -ACC-, another codon for threonine. Then he removed the -ACT- codon for threonine and replaced it with -TCT-, another codon for serine. Thus he switched the Ser[70]-Thr[71] sequence to Thr[70]-Ser[71].

The research team then spliced this human-mutated gene into a plasmid inside *E. coli,* bred about a billion of the bacteria and collected the beta-lactamase they made. The enzyme, which normally destroys penicillin, turned out to be totally inactive. Richards had succeeded in modifying a gene to make a specialized biological product. The implications for biotechnology are, of course, immense. Custom-designed drugs, enzymes, vitamins and peptides—including novel forms of endorphins—are no longer the stuff of science fiction. What Richards did with beta-lactamase in a petri dish will someday be done with endorphin in multi-liter fermentation vats.

Some Possibilities

Just what will happen in the future is hard to say. As Table 11.1 points out, even the most likely candidates for biotech-produced products are still several years in the future. Some we may well not see on the marketplace until near the turn of the century. Endorphins and other opioid peptides aren't even included in the table, because the source company, Genex, still doesn't see a likely commercial breakthrough for them.

Given their potential, though, and the range of possible physiological and medical connections, we can be pretty sure that endorphins will someday be commercially available. Their likely involvement in pain suppression, mental illness, drug addiction, learning and memory and other processes makes the business of endorphins a near certainty. How near that certainty is—that is still the sixty-four-dollar question. But even the less likely endorphin connections, if proven in some small way, could lead to commercial use of the opioid peptides.

Consider, for example, the possible endorphin/arthritis connection. Charles Denko's experiments showed that people suffering from rheumatoid arthritis have lower than normal levels of endorphins in their blood and joint fluids. People afflicted with the especially painful and crippling versions of this disease have especially low levels of the peptide. This isn't proof of a causal connection between the two, much less proof that low endorphin levels are the cause and arthritis the effect. There's more work to be done. But what if that connection turned out to be true? Yes, aspirin works to relieve the inflammation in the less severe cases, and so do some other anti-inflammatory agents like naproxen and ibuprofen. Local injections of certain corticosteroids can be effective for up to three weeks, but long-term use has undesirable side effects. And none of these treatments results in a cure, but only an alleviation of the symptoms.

Simply on the level of a pain-killer, endorphins might be quite effective. We already know they effectively and swiftly relieve the pain of terminal cancer patients and women in labor. They don't act in the brain in those cases because they don't have to; the analgesic activity takes place in the pain-transmission nerves in the spinal cord. In the case of painful rheumatoid arthritis, this too could be the case. The pain may result from lower than normal endorphin levels caused by the arthritis. In that case, endorphin injections into the affected areas could well control the pain swiftly and for a long time. Or, the endorphin deficiency could be part of the cause of rheumatoid arthritis. If that is indeed the case, endorphin injections would be more than just a way to relieve the symptoms; they could result in arresting or even curing the affliction.

Again, a warning: none of this is known to be true. But it is a possibility. The point is, if either of these scenarios turn out to be true, someone is going to make a buck from it. Endorphins will go commercial. Can we visualize the ads? "Endorf-Away! *The* way to banish the aches and pains of arthritis and bursitis!!!"

Endorphins for Mental Illness

Determining the future of endorphins and mental illness is next to impossible at this point. Still too little is truly known of the links between these opiate peptides and the tragic afflictions of manic-depression, catatonia, paranoid schizophrenia and the galaxy of other mental illnesses that plague more than six and a half million Americans.

But we can make some reasonable guesses, based on what we do know. The cumulated evidence of animal experimentation and clinical trials suggests that levels of endorphins and endorphin-like compounds are somehow connected to one or more forms of schizophrenia. There may well be a connection involving DTgE, the endorphin-like fragment that actually has no opiate-like activity. And the evidence for the "dopamine excess theory" does make considerable sense when looked at in relation to DTgE. It's also very likely that the real connection involves some intricate balance in the brain among endorphins, dynorphin, DTgE, dopamine and probably acetylcholine and norepinephrine as well.

Then we have the intriguing results of electroconvulsive shock experiments on rats. It does indeed seem that Met-enkephalin levels in the brain have some important connection with how that master organ regulates our emotions. That in turn certainly has something to do with the powerful emotional component of so many mental afflictions.

Almost from the beginning of endorphin research it has been possible to make synthetic versions of the opiate peptides, and even new variations of them that don't exist in nature. Today, companies like Smith-Kline Beckman, Genentech, and Peninsula Laboratories near San Francisco make synthetic endorphins in large enough quantities to sell to various researchers. Eventually —and perhaps sooner than we think—companies such as these will master the technology for making synthetic opioid peptides in commercially salable quantities. If something like DTgE proves to be an effective treatment for some form of mental illness, it could be the beginning of a whole new industry.

So what might the future hold? I think it's likely we will see, before the turn of the century, a new form of drug therapy for mentally ill people. We will see the disappearance from the psychiatric tool kit of neuroleptic drugs like haloperidol and Thorazine®, with their tragic long-term side effects. Instead, doctors will use endorphins to treat the mentally ill. Some of the chemicals they use will be commercially produced, in much the same way genetic engineering companies have begun producing human insulin on a giant scale for diabetics. Some of these synthetic endorphins will be identical to the ones our brains and bodies produce. Others will be different from "the natural thing," tailored to be more powerful, or more gentle, or more specific in action. ("Just the amygdala, Doctor; this lady's got a severe emotional disorder.")

And some patients may well be treated with their own endorphins, extracted under local anesthetic (which may itself be an endorphin!) from their cerebrospinal fluid during routine checkup visits and held in reserve for moments of mental crisis.

The best form of medicine, though, is preventive. And this, too, will someday be possible with endorphins. Unborn infants will undergo placental fluid analyses that will show whether or not they are genetically and biochemically "at risk" when it comes to mental illness. The same kind of tests are being done today, to determine if the fetuses have Rh blood problems, or if they have the chromosomal abnormalities that can give rise to Down's syndrome, sickle-cell anemia and other genetically caused problems. And just as some conditions today can be treated *in utero,* so these kinds might be dealt with in the near future. Unborn fetuses may receive infusions of ultra-minute quantities of chemicals to increase or decrease the levels of endorphins in their tiny brains. Imbalances can be corrected before they cause problems—before the child is even born.

And as these infants get older, they can if necessary receive preventive doses of naloxone-like antagonists or endorphin-like peptides to keep the specter of mental illness far from the doors of their psyches.

The age of mental hospitals and of the palsied "walking wounded" of outpatient clinics will come to an end. And a new age of care and treatment for the mentally ill will begin.

The Underground Economy

Finally, we shouldn't neglect the real possibility of the criminalization of endorphins. Such a thing may seem pretty farfetched at first glance. Endorphins, if they are to have any powerful addictive effects, must be administered into the central nervous system. The blood-brain barrier prevents most opioid peptides injected into the bloodstream from getting into the brain. That would seem to make it highly unlikely that anyone could get addicted to beta-endorphin in the same way a person gets addicted to heroin. The method of administration for smack just won't work for opioid peptides, and it's difficult to imagine anyone performing an intrathecal or intraventricular injection on oneself.

If we think that's the end of it, we're fooling ourselves. People can give each other such injections, if they wish, and if they have steady enough hands. Ask any junkie about how rock-steady one gets when it's time to shoot up. Then there's the fact that the BBB isn't perfect. While it filters out almost all of an intravenously administered opioid peptide, it doesn't stop all of it. Such a peptide could be reengineered for extreme addictive potency. Even taken into the body intravenously it could be so potent that just a few hundred nanomoles sneaking through the BBB would be enough to cause addiction.

We mentioned earlier in the book that some researchers have found ways to redesign drugs so they can more easily slip through the blood-brain barrier into the brain. It's already been done with a chemical similar to dopamine. It probably won't be much longer before it can—and will—be done for an endorphin-type peptide.

If such scenarios came true, it is not beyond the realm of possibility that another would, also: the one at the beginning of Chapter 7. The passage of anti-drug laws depends heavily on the sociopolitical climate of the times. In the 1930s it was marijuana; in the 1960s it was LSD. Perhaps in the 1990s it will be "Enkephalin Z." And with that, as with the others, will come a flourishing *underground* business in illicit endorphins. Science fiction writers, take note!

Nor need the situation be so extreme. Librium®, Valium® and Percodan® are perfectly legal drugs. One needs a prescription to get them, of course. And of course that doesn't even put a dent in their massive abuse in this country. It is not at all difficult to imagine a similar situation with "prescription-only" Enkefordan® or Dynilium®.

* * *

If there is a dark side to the coming endorphin revolution, it is because there is a dark side to us. We have to wonder at times why we insist on doing these things to ourselves; why we have this perverse penchant for taking technologies with marvelous possibilities for healing and turning them into instruments of evil and death. It's a question for which our science and technologies do not have an answer.

TABLE 11.1
FUTURE BIOTECH PRODUCTS

Product	U.S. market, 1981 (tons/year)	Commercialization (year)
Amino acids		
Glutamate	300,000	1988
Methionine	105,000	1993
Lysine	64,500	1988
Aspartate	1,500	1988
Vitamins		
Vitamin C	45,000	1993
Vitamin E	1,820	1998
Nicotinic acid	700	1993
Enzymes		
Bacillus protease	500	1988
Amylglucosidase	300	1988
Glucose isomerase	50	1988
Hormones		
Prednisone	—	1993
Testosterone	—	1993
Estradiol	—	1993
Human growth hormone	—	1988
Vasopressin	—	1988

Based on data from Genex Corp., as published in *High Technology*, February 1983.

12

Beyond Endorphins

"Paradigm" is a fancy word for "model." When scientists use it, they usually mean a really big model, something even bigger than a hypothesis or theory. A paradigm is a world view, a framework into which hypotheses and theories fit like pictures.

The current brain paradigm sees that organ as one that is electrobiochemically powered, with strong overtones of holographic storage. This paradigm has come into play in the last several decades as scientists have learned more and more about the brain's actual operation. The key to that operation is the complex interaction of chemicals in the brain. The deeper the scientists and researchers get into the operation of the human brain, the more complex and puzzling it gets and the more intricate the interactions of the dozens—probably hundreds—of chemicals within.

Another paradigm has to do with our view of the nature of reality itself. That paradigm is still in the process of changing, and part of that change is in our view of the relationship between the brain and what we call the mind.

So we'll look at several things in this final chapter: the likelihood of discovering new brain chemicals beyond the opioid peptides, and of determining their role in the brain's operation; the paradigms for brain-mind interaction; and the emerging new paradigm for reality, and how it affects our understanding of brain, and mind, and the function of endorphins. There is something refreshing about throwing caution to the wind. We will.

New Brain Chemicals?

Any new chemicals we discover in the brain are not really "new"; they've been there all along. It's our knowledge of them that's new. With that caveat in mind, we can say pretty confidently that neuropharmacologists and brain biologists will find chemicals in the brain which we do not now know exist. They'll be found for the same reasons and in the same way the endorphins were found: evidential fingers point to their existence; and labeling, staining, protein synthesis and DNA cloning techniques will find them.

Consider the matter of marijuana, *Cannabis sativa*. The active ingredient in marijuana is called THC, or tetrahydrocannabinol. It produces euphoric effects when it's eaten or smoked and is usually classified as a hallucinogen. Marijuana preparations are also being used experimentally to treat the symptoms of glaucoma, an eye disease characterized by a radical increase in the eye fluid's internal pressure, sometimes severe pain and eventually blindness. It seems to work. Question: why do these things happen? What's going on in the brain when THC hits the neurons and their synapses? *Why* does it cause euphoric effects? What neurotransmitter system is it interacting with? And why does it seem to alleviate some of the symptoms associated with severe cases of glaucoma? What's the connection there?

As of this writing we don't have the answers to these questions. The answers do exist. There must be a connection between the effects of marijuana and the brain's neurotransmitter system. Marijuana causes distortions of our emotions, of our physical responses to external and internal stimuli, and of our perception of reality. All these activities arise in and are modulated by different parts of the brain. All these activities have their origins in the actions and interactions of different neurotransmission systems. The THC in marijuana is doing something to those systems. What? Most likely, plugging into some kind of neuronal receptor site. Which one? At this point, no one knows. But certainly that receptor site did not evolve solely for the pleasure of marijuana-eating or -smoking creatures. The receptor that THC plugs into is in the brain for other purposes. Just as the operation of external opiates pointed to the existence of internal opioids, so the action of THC points to the existence of some internal brain chemical with similar properties. What is it? What's it there for?

The answers are not far off. A number of researchers are working to find it, among them Candace Pert, the co-discoverer of the opiate receptor. By the time you have this in your hand, she or some other scientist may well have found "marijuana receptors" in the brain of some laboratory rat or guinea pig. Or perhaps even in the brain of a human being.

That in turn will eventually lead to the discovery of endogenous "THC-like" chemicals. And that will lead to the explanation of the effects marijuana has on glaucoma symptoms. Eventually we may see other THC connections in the brain to our behavior and perceptions.

If this scenario sounds like the actual history of the discovery of endorphins, good. It's supposed to. That's one way the discoveries of brain chemicals beyond endorphins will happen. It will also happen serendipitously, by surprise, by accident. That's the way researchers in 1982 discovered the existence and location of appetite receptors in the brain.

The researchers were Steven M. Paul and Bridget Hulihan-Giblin of the National Institute of Mental Health (NIMH) and Phil Skolnick of the National Institute of Arthritis, Diabetes and Digestive and Kidney Diseases. The three had an interest in the biochemical basis of seizures, psychoses and anxiety, and so they naturally had an interest in the actions of amphetamines, which can and do cause such conditions. In both humans and laboratory animals amphetamines also cause increased motor activity. The researchers set out to find where in the brain amphetamines might be binding to neuron receptor sites. Surprisingly, they found amphetamines binding to two places that had nothing at all to do with motor activity. One site was on nerve endings in the hypothalamus and lower brain stem. Paul and Skolnick found that the ability of amphetamines and related chemicals to bind to these sites was directly related to their ability to suppress appetite. The researchers had found the receptors in the brain that specifically regulate appetite suppression.

Brain scientists have pointed to a number of different neurotransmitters which might be involved in the regulation of appetite: epinephrine, norepinephrine, dopamine and serotonin are most often mentioned. Skolnick and Paul think the appetite-suppressing receptors to which amphetamines bind are probably release sites for norepinephrine or serotonin, but that's still not proven.

The discovery of opiate receptors led to the discovery of the endorphins. Could the discovery of the appetite receptors lead to the finding of "endogenous amphetamines," which the brain uses in its natural regulation of appetite? It's possible. It's also possible the situation is a lot more complex than one receptor for this one function. Certainly the serotoninergic and NE-ergic systems interact, and they could be doing so to effect the control of appetite. It's still too early to tell. But the implications are intriguing. We may yet wake up one morning to find that Paul and Skolnick, or some other researchers, have found and identified "endophetamines."

The sigma receptor presents another puzzle. Does it exist? Some say it is the one with which a benzomorph drug called SKF-10,047 interacts. Other researchers claim that PCP interacts with the sigma receptor. But is it really something separate? Or is the "sigma receptor" perhaps a subtype of the more well-known kappa receptor, the receptor for dynorphin?

And what about the endorphins themselves? Have we reached an end to them? Have we found all of the endogenous opioid peptides which exist in the brain and body?

Not likely. Not yet. There's little likelihood we will find any more endorphins proper. Beta-endorphin and its fragments are fully accounted for in the POMC precursor protein. However, the adrenal medulla seems to be the source of a plethora of enkephalin-like peptides of various sizes. We probably haven't found all of those yet. And then there are the dynorphins. Researchers have found at least a half-dozen in the brain—dynorphin-8, -13, -24, -32, -A and -B—as well as alpha-neo-endorphin, which is related to the dynorphins through the pre-prodynorphin precursor. There don't seem to be any more opioid peptides lurking in pre-prodynorphin, but the Japanese discoverers did suggest some may still be found.

And dynorphin remains a bit of a puzzle. It shows opiate activity in many tests, but recent research also shows it has non-opiate activity as well. And many of its actions in the body are just the opposite of those of the other endorphins. Narcotics and endorphins increase the firing rate of the pyramidal neurons in the hippocampus, but dynorphin inhibits them. Beta-endorphin induces sedation and catatonic-like postures in rats; dynorphin causes strange, contorted postures. And while many of the changes caused in experimental animals by endorphins are reversed or stopped by injections of naloxone, those caused by dynorphin are not. Obviously, dynorphin plays a role not only in an opiate pathway in the brain, as the other endorphins do, but also in a non-opiate pathway. What is that pathway? What are its locations and receptor sites? What does it do for the body? Also, the dynorphin precursor has a large section of nucleotides that hasn't yet been decoded. It could include other dynorphin-type peptides, or perhaps opioid peptides we still don't know about.

The existence and structure of the opioid precursors also raise questions reaching beyond endorphins—questions connected with the process of biological and biochemical evolution. The opiate precursors are all remarkably similar in size. POMC has 265 amino acids; pre-proenkephalin, 267; and pre-prodynorphin, 256 amino acids. They all have "signal peptides" at their beginnings which are similar in length, about twenty or so amino acids long. They each have six serines in them which form disulfide bonds, causing the molecules to fold over for efficient processing into their component endorphins. They all have repeating internal sequences of nucleotides in their genetic codes. This all suggests that the three precursors themselves evolved from a common DNA ancestor. It could well have occurred more than a billion years ago, since Candace Pert and others have already found endorphin-like chemicals in one-celled creatures that have been on earth at least that long. And the repeated internal sequences of nucleotides seem to indicate that a particular part of the gene was duplicated over and over again. These and other pieces of information about the structure of the endorphin precursors and their DNA codes will lead to further unravelings of the evolutionary history of the brain and its chemical structure.

We certainly still have a lot to do to confirm or deny some of the possible roles for endorphins in the brain and body. For one thing, are they *really* neurotransmitters? Everything seems to suggest they are. But although we've referred to them as such throughout this book, they are more accurately called "putative neurotransmitters." Actually *proving* an endorphin is a neurotransmitter is pretty difficult. First we'd have to retrieve some of the fluid surrounding some brain neurons and some of that in the synaptic gap, and we'd have to retrieve it after a neuron has fired off a signal to the next one in line. Then we'd have to find out if there was any of the opioid peptide in the fluid, and we'd have to prove it wasn't there before the neuron fired. Then we'd have to remove the peptide from the fluid and re-inject it into the synaptic gap of two neurons which are not firing off. And *then* we'd have to see if this caused the postsynaptic neuron to fire off.

And if that occurs we'll have to do the same again, and again and again, to eliminate any chances of extraneous interference and to get some good statistical probabilities on our experiment.

And then at least one or two other researchers in other labs should do the same experiment, with the same types of equipment, and get the same results. This all takes a lot of time and a lot of money and a lot of effort. And it has never been done, for *any* "putative neurotransmitter." In the end we are all basing our identification of acetylcholine, dopamine, epinephrine, serotonin, GABA, Substance P and the endorphins as neurotransmitters on purely circumstantial evidence.

Perhaps, in the future, some researchers will get enough money and time so they can definitely prove, one way or another, that endorphins are neurotransmitters. Perhaps.

One area that will certainly come into clearer focus in the next few years will be the methods of interaction of the different opioid systems in the brain—with each other as well as with other neurotransmitter systems. We now know that the enkephalins, beta-endorphin and the dynorphins comprise separate neuronal pathway systems in the brain. We know they overlap in some areas, too. What does that overlapping mean? How do they interact in these areas, or do they? And why are the three systems for the most part separate? What is the purpose of that? The answers to these questions are intimately tied to the elucidation of the various endorphin connections with physiological and mental states of the human being. As we learn more about those connections, as we discover which are real and which are merely experimental or logical artifacts, we will also learn more about how the different endorphin chemicals interact in the brain and body.

Endorphins and Meditation

Is meditation a form of addiction, as some might suggest? Or is it a legitimate method of trying to make contact with realities beyond the one we inhabit—this reality of matter and energy? Probably both. And in either case endorphins might play a role. The opioid peptides are addictive. And they do play some kind of role in opiate addiction. We've also seen, more to the point, that they are inhibitory chemicals which can slow down the firing of certain neuronal systems and impart a feeling of calm, relaxation, and being "naturally high." These are characteristic psychological states associated with certain forms of deep or contemplative meditation, including TM, Zen and Centering Prayer. Whether or not the person doing the meditating is "in contact" with another reality or simply doing something in her/his brain, the brain *is* involved, and the body *is* involved. For that reason alone we can legitimately speculate that endorphins and other opioid peptides may well be playing some kind of role in meditative states.

Sometimes the person meditating will experience other psychological states, akin to Goldstein's "thrills." Those too may be connected with the operation of endogenous opioid peptides.

All of which leads in some roundabout way to the matter of mind and brain.

Mind and Brain: Two or One?

For hundreds of years now philosophers have been coming to metaphorical blows over the question of mind and brain. Are they the same, or different? Our ever-increasing understanding of how the brain works has not served to settle the question, but only to intensify the argument.

Basically, there are two ways of looking at the mind-brain question: the mind and the brain are two separate and distinct entities which interact with each other to some degree; or, the mind and the brain are one and the same, and dualistic perceptions about them are illusory. Most scientists today probably consider themselves materialists and positivists, and so would subscribe to the latter concept. Materialism is a philosophy which states that matter alone is real, nothing else. So mental phenomena, including the mind, are all products of material phenomena. The operation of the brain creates mind. Indeed, the mind is nothing more than the ongoing operation of the incredibly complex organ inside our skulls. Positivism is a philosophy which contends that sense impressions are the only admissible basis for knowledge and precise thought. Logical positivism, a variation of this, asserts the primacy of observation in assessing the truth of statements of fact, arguments not based on observable data are meaningless. To talk about the mind as a nonmaterial entity separate from the brain (whether or not it interacts with that organ) is simply meaningless babble to the materialist or logical positivist.

One of contemporary science's greatest champions of mind-body unity was Gregory Bateson, the anthropologist. In much of his writing he asserted his strongly held belief that the mind and the brain were not two but one. "Mental processes do not exist until matter reaches certain degrees of organization," he said in a dialogue with Dr. Robert Reiber in *Body and Mind: Past, Present and Future,* edited by Reiber. Shortly afterwards he added: "Mind is no more separate from body than velocity is separate from matter. Or than acceleration is separate from velocity."

Bateson is not alone in his monistic paradigm of mind and brain. It's a stance that's easy and comfortable for many to take, especially scientists. For science deals with matter/energy and its interactions. It does not, *by definition,* deal with anything which is not matter/energy. If mind is neither matter nor energy, nor a product of matter/energy interactions, then science cannot deal with it. And scientists can't deal with it scientifically.

However, the dualistic concepts of mind and brain are not without either pedigree or defenders. In fact, science itself originates in part from the dualistic world view of the famous philosopher/mathematician/scientist René Descartes (1596–1650). Descartes asserted the belief that the observer (you and I) and the observed (the rest of the universe) are distinct and separate, a concept which makes science as we know it today possible. He also said that the mind and the brain (the senses) are separate, and that God is the mediator between the two.

One of the most important advocates of a dualistic concept of mind and brain was the late Dr. Wilder Penfield, the famous neurosurgeon. In a series of pioneering operations on epileptics which he began in the 1930s, Penfield discovered the location in the brain of many of our "mental" processes. He performed hundreds of operations over several decades. The people remained conscious (the brain has no sense receptors in it, so it feels no pain) and could relate to him what they were feeling, experiencing and remembering as he delicately probed their brains with electrodes. One thing Penfield never found—nor has anyone else—was a discrete location for "the mind." He finally reached the conclusion that the mind simply was not present in the brain. However, he did think there was a place in the brain where mind interacted with it. That place is the supplementary motor area, or SMA, which Penfield discovered in 1943. The SMA is located in both the left and the right brain hemispheres, on their upper mid-surface just underneath the skull.

In recent years a series of experiments have shown powerful indications of the SMA's role in the control of all voluntary movement, and even in the *attempted* control of such movement in paralyzed people. These experiments were done using a brain-scanning technique called PET, which stands for positron-emission tomography. It creates a fifteen-color mosaic map of a living human brain and shows which parts are in activity from moment to moment. Researchers in Denmark, Australia, Germany and other places have used this and other techniques to show there is evidence that the mind acts *on the brain,* and does so *in a specific area of the cortex.* Penfield's theory of the role of the SMA now seems to be proving true.

Two other contemporary champions of mind-brain dualism are the philosopher Sir Karl Popper and the Nobel Prize-winning neurobiologist Sir John Eccles. They have proposed and refined a version of this idea which they call "dualistic interactionism." This concept holds that humans live in two distinct worlds, the material world (what Popper calls "World 1") and the world of mental processes and consciousness (or "World 2"). There is an intense and continual interplay between these two worlds, and out of it arises a third world, "World 3," the world of knowledge in all its forms—science, philosophy, religion, literature and art. Humans store traces of World 3 in sections of World 1: in books, paintings, sculpture, film and ritual; and in memory tracks in the human brain.

Which brain-mind paradigm is closest to the truth is not possible to determine. We don't know nearly enough about the brain yet to hazard more than what we already have: hypotheses and guesses. In both cases, though, neurotransmitters like the endorphins play an important role. We've seen how these opioid peptides are implicated in the perception of pain, in mental illness, in the abuse of and addiction to chemicals which alter reality perceptions, and in a number of other physical and mental conditions. Endorphins are intimately involved in our perception, interaction with and control of "the world outside."

Perhaps the mind is something separate from the brain, which acts in the world of matter/energy through interaction with that organ. Endorphins then play a crucial role in that interaction, assisting in the mediation of the mind's coupling with the brain through the SMA to deeper brain regions. Remember, endorphins are like GABA, an inhibitory neurochemical. Without their action to slow down neuronal firing, the racing electrical storms of activity would result in bodily convulsions and death.

Perhaps mind isn't separate from brain, but instead something created by the brain's activity itself. The mind is what philosophers call an "epiphenomenon," a secondary phenomenon created by and dependent on a primary phenomenon. Endorphins, then, play a crucial role in the very creation of that epiphenomenon, in the existence and operation of the mind.

The Emerging Reality Paradigm

There is an ancient Chinese curse: "May you live in interesting times." And if such is true, then we are indeed accursed. One of the things making our times so interesting is the imminent shift in our reality paradigm. It's been coming on for more than eighty years now. It began at nearly the same moment as the current paradigm of the brain, in the last year of the nineteenth century (though common belief makes it the first year of the twentieth).

On December 14, 1900, quantum physics was born, fathered (and mothered) by Max Planck. For most of the century the consequences of quantum physics have remained unknown to the average person. Oh, we have radio and television and nuclear bombs and lasers and a myriad other devices and inventions whose very existence depends on the truth of quantum physics. But most of us didn't know that. Now, more and more of us are becoming aware of the philosophical implications of a theory of reality put together eighty-four years ago in a fit of utter desperation.

By the end of the nineteenth century, "classical physics" found itself in a hopeless bind. Scientists were doing experiments and coming up with results, and finding that their predictions of those results, based on the physics of Isaac Newton, were not the same as the results themselves. This was not just some irritating little glitch. It was an unmitigated disaster. It meant that the world view they'd been using all this time was *wrong,* or at best incomplete.

The response to this impasse was twofold: Albert Einstein invented the special theory of relativity, and Max Planck invented the idea of the quantum. Einstein's theory was not so much a break with classic Newtonian physics as it was a culmination of it. Newton's physics didn't become false, but only a "special case" in the larger picture of relativistic physics. Relativity, like all classical physics up to that date, had built into it the logical and common-sense assumption that *there is such a thing as an objective world "out there,"* and that *it is separate and distinct from the objective world "in here"*—that is, me. The observer, in other words, is separate from what is observed, and both are real. In fact, all of science rests on the assumption that we can speak of an objective reality, a reality apart from ourselves, a reality we can observe and test without interfering with it.

Planck's idea of the quantum was that energy comes in discrete "packages" rather than in continuously flowing "waves," and that those "packages" sometimes acted as if they were sometimes particles and sometimes waves. It was a total break with classical physics. It meant the universe could not ultimately be seen as a collection of tiny "things" floating in space and interacting in precise patterns. Physicists and mathematicians following Planck elaborated on his idea, and showed that everything could be described by complex mathematical terms called "quantum wave functions," or QWFs. A QWF was not a "thing" at all, not a wave or a particle or a particle-wave or anything. It was a probability of something.

As the century progressed and various physicists explored the new theory's ramifications, some very disturbing consequences began to appear. Werner Heisenberg stated one of those disturbing consequences in his famous "Principle of Uncertainty." We can't perform an experiment without interfering—even in the tiniest way—with the results. Over and over again, this proved true. No matter how careful we are in setting up our experiments, we find we disturb the experiment by doing the experiment. Experiments are just special ways of observing reality. If Heisenberg's Uncertainty Principle is true in those cases, it's true in all cases. It comes down to this: *the observer and the observed are not separate.* The observer is an individual using his or her mind (whatever that is) to observe "Nature." In attempting to observe, though, mind interacts with what is observed—that is, the cosmos. Mind is not separate from what mind observes. In observing, the mind of the observer "collapses" all the possible QWFs from a probability to a certainty.

Does this seem outrageous? Of course it does. It goes against common sense and common experience. The moon hasn't changed just because I've looked at it! I pick up an orange and smell it. Has the orange changed because I smelled it? Of course not!

Wrong, says quantum physics. The moon *has* been changed by your observation. The orange *is* different because you smelled it. You may not sense the changes, because your sensory apparatus is too coarse to sense it. In fact, if you could sense the change, that sensing would change the change! It may be outrageous and insane-sounding. But there's one thing scientists respect—*must* respect—and that's results. Quantum physics gives results, and the results of this theory are better than those of any other. For more than fifty years scientists have tried to come up with substitutes for or modifications of quantum physics that can do just as good a job of predicting the results of experiments. None has worked as well as quantum physics itself. *None.*

The theory of the quantum says the dualism of observer and observed is an illusion. I and the universe are one. Literally. Yet we are also separate in the sense that I *sense* myself as separate from it. Everything seems somewhat magical and strange and weird, when you think about it this way. Of course, if we were Taoists or Buddhists none of this would be strange at all. It would be part of our world view, our paradigm. But we're Westerners, and it's new and strange and very uncomfortable. For a lot of scientists it's simply intolerable. So they just don't think about the implications.

Endorphins and the Quantum

The connection between endorphins, quantum physics and the mind and brain is not just a product of logic: "Quantum physics is connected to everything; endorphins are part of everything; everything includes the mind and the brain; therefore quantum physics is connected to endorphins and the mind and the brain." There is a real connection; "real" as in "operative," as in "this happens in the 'real world' of the human brain." In some bizarre yet real way we make the universe exist by observing it. We collapse a QWF representing a possible state for an electron (left spin or right spin?) by observing it. But quantum physics does not, cannot if it is true, just apply to subatomic physics. It must apply to everything. So we also collapse the QWF representing a light (on or off) by opening the door to the room and looking in. Does mind therefore make endorphins real? If so, how? How does mind make the process of synaptic neurotransmission work? What mind is collapsing the QWFs that could potentially be endorphins plugging into receptors, and electrical waves racing down neurons? In trying to see how it might apply to endorphins, we see that quantum physics casts new light on the old question of brain-mind dualism, and on the two possible answers to that question.

If the human mind is a part of World 2 separate from the brain, as Popper and Eccles suggest, then it can collapse the endorphin QWFs, dynorphin QWFs, enkephalin QWFs, receptor site on/off QWFs, and all the other QWFs of World 1 that lead to a wave of electrical potential either passing or not passing down a neuron.

In this case, endorphins remain pretty much as we think of them now: products of the brain and endocrine systems. The mind works through and in concert with the brain, possibly via the SMA region; endorphins and other neurotransmitters/hormones are essential to that interaction. Without them, the brain does not work. Reality (whatever *that* is) cannot be perceived.

However, this doesn't explain the *mind*—or anything else which is a part of Popper's World 2. The human mind may be happily opening all those quantum boxes and collapsing all those QWFs into endorphins, closed or open receptor sites, polarized or depolarized cell membranes, and so on. But what makes the human mind? How do *its* QWFs get collapsed?

In his book *Taking the Quantum Leap,* physicist Fred Alan Wolf suggests that what we call "mind" is a property of all matter/energy, right down to peptides, atoms, electrons and quarks. It's a simple mind, this molecular or atomic or quarkish mind. It can make simple yes/no decisions, on/off choices. Does this electron have a clockwise or counterclockwise spin? The position of the two hydrogen atoms in the NH_2- terminal of this molecule of Met-enkephalin—up or down? The atomic minds choose. They choose randomly. Up—the molecule fits into the receptor site and the membrane is inhibited. Down—the molecule doesn't plug in, the membrane is that much closer to depolarizing. The molecule's "mind" will make the random choice. For one particular neuron, receiving hundreds of potential signals from hundreds of other neurons every millisecond, all those decisions by all those molecules of beta-endorphin—plus all the thousands of other potential inputs from other neurotransmitter molecules—will add up to one of two possibilities. Either the membrane will be so depolarized as to fire off an electrical wave, or it won't. One way or the other, the "yes/no" decisions of all the neurotransmitters will lead to the collapse of the QWF representing the "on/off" state of the neuron. Every instant, that QWF collapses into "fire" or "not-fire". And that happens *every instant for every single one of the hundred-billion-plus neurons in the brain.*

Remember those big numbers we talked about at the very beginning of the book? Each of the hundred-billion-plus neurons has an average of a thousand connections with other neurons, and that means there are at least one hundred trillion interconnections. And *that* means there are $2^{100,000,000,000,000}$ possible states for the human brain to be in. Instant by instant, $2^{100,000,000,000,000}$ QWFs get collapsed in the 1400-gram mass of cells inside our skulls. All of it happening through the yes/no decision of atomic/molecular minds. And all those choices, by all those molecular and atomic minds, combine synergistically to create what I call "my" mind, "my" sense of self-awareness and self-consciousness.

Is it true? Are we really nothing more than an epiphenomenon of atomic minds? Or is there something nonmaterial, non-World 1, which interacts with the brain of World 1 and so creates World 1?

We don't know. And we may never know. We will certainly not know through the efforts of science. For science cannot answer questions or study phenomena which are not rooted in the reality of matter/energy (World 1). Even when it has itself proved that that reality is nothing more than a shadow cast by the minds which observe it.

Beyond Endorphins

We began this book in the realm of atoms and molecules; moved on to the level of brain structures and activities, bodily functions and dysfunctions; got as far as capitalistic economics; and ended up at a level below the one where we started, at the level of quantum wave functions and the existence of the mind.

It's been a long, strange trip, as the Grateful Dead's Jerry Garcia once sang. We did it with our brains, and with the chemicals in our brains. In fact, if endorphins have anything at all to do with memory and learning then we did it with the help of the very peptides this book is about.

But this trip has really just begun. As I write these final words, it's 8:30 P.M., Pacific Standard Time, March 20, 1983: the beginning of spring in Terra's northern hemisphere. Ten years and eleven days ago Candace Pert and Solomon Snyder announced they had demonstrated the existence of opiate receptors in brain tissue. It was the beginning of a new wave of understanding in brain chemistry. More than a decade later, we have answered some questions; we still search for the answers to others; we've found many more to seek answers to; and we find ourselves wondering if some of the deepest questions we ask can ever be answered.

Perhaps. Perhaps not. But as long as the vesicles pop, the neurotransmitters flow and the nerve cells fire, we'll keep looking. And who knows what we'll find beyond endorphins?

AFTERWORD

Recent Developments

Writing a book on a scientific subject can be risky. One reason is that things always change, and in science things can change very quickly. A popular book on astronomy written in late 1962 and published a year later—a time lag less than the one this book has experienced—would have been obsolete when it hit the bookstores. Quasars were discovered between the time it was written and the time it was published.

The problem can be even worse for a book on biochemistry—specifically for a book on endorphins. The entire field of endorphin science didn't even exist twelve years ago. Since that time the endogenous opioid peptides have been discovered, categorized, synthesized and tested in human beings. Dozens of actual and possible endorphin connections have been examined, and we have looked at some of those connections in the pages of this book.

The initial manuscript for *Endorphins: New Waves in Brain Chemistry* was finished on March 20, 1983. Science has not stood still in the months since then. A computer search of the National Library of Medicine's data base, using the search term "endorphins," produced a list of 397 citations for articles published between January 1 and November 23, 1983. That's a rate of more than one scientific report on endorphins per day! I did a manual search and came up with another half-dozen endorphin reports published in December 1983 and the first couple of weeks in 1984.

Now, most of those papers dealt with the minutiae of laboratory experimentation typical of most scientific work. Very little of the science done by scientists is pathbreaking. Most of it is follow-up and follow-through. Nevertheless, a number of interesting (Mr. Spock might even say fascinating) results emerged from research on endorphins in the last year. Herewith, a quick sampling to make this book as up-to-date as possible.

In Chapter 3, "The Discovery of Endorphins," we detailed the sequence of events involved in the discovery of the endogenous opioid peptides. In Chapter 5, "The Endogenous Opioid Peptides," we took a close look at the nature of the endorphins, enkephalins and dynorphins we know exist. In the last year several new opioid peptides have been discovered.

In May of 1983, Sydney Spector and his colleagues at the Roche Institute for Molecular Biology in New Jersey announced that they had developed monoclonal antibodies for morphine. They found that these antibodies do not bind to any of the known opioid peptides—not too surprising, since morphine is a much larger molecule than the endorphins, and has for the most part a considerably different chemical structure.

However, later in the year Spector found that his morphine monoclonal antibodies *did* bind to three chemicals found in extracts of beef brain. At least one of the chemicals has three times the affinity for opiate receptors as does morphine—in other words, it is a previously undiscovered opioid peptide. As of this writing, this new "endorphin" has not yet been fully characterized. Nor does anyone know its natural function in the brain.

Two other new opioid peptides have been discovered in living creatures, and they have been fully characterized and named. One is called *adrenorphin*, and its discovery was reported by Hisayuki Matsuo (a familiar name from Chapters 3 and 5) and his colleagues in Japan. Adrenorphin was found in a tumor which came from the medulla of a human adrenal gland. This opioid peptide has eight amino acids in it. It is "written" like this:

Tyr-Gly-Gly-Phe-Met-Arg-Arg-Val

Adrenorphin's first five amino acids, of course, are identical to Met-enkephalin. The adrenorphin sequence is found in the huge precursor molecule for the enkephalins named pre-proenkephalin. It runs from positions 210 to 217. The valine in position eight is followed in pre-proenkephalin by glycine, arginine and proline. When adrenorphin is split out of pre-proenkephalin, the glycine is replaced by NH_2. What's puzzling, though, is the Arg-Pro amino acid pair, which is not known to be a standard processing signal.

Adrenorphin has a dynorphin near-twin: dynorphin-8 has a leucine instead of a methionine, and ilene instead of valine. Dynorphin-8, of course, is found in pre-prodynorphin (also known as pre-proenkephalin B). And it is in almost exactly the same position in the dynorphin precursor, positions 209–216, as adrenorphin is in its precursor.

As far as opiate potency is concerned, adrenorphin is fifteen times as powerful as Met-enkephalin in the standard tests. The enkephalin-containing peptide (ECP) known as BAM-12P has glycine, arginine, proline and glutamic acid following the adrenorphin sequence. However, BAM-12P is only one fifth as potent as adrenorphin.

The other new opioid peptide discovered in 1983 is called *leumorphin*.

Leumorphin was in a sense "discovered" back in 1982, as the last part of the pre-prodynorphin (pre-proenkephalin B) precursor molecule. We talked about pre-prodynorphin's structure in Chapter 5, and there mentioned the third Leu-enkephalin at its end (positions 228–232). That third Leu-enkephalin is followed by twenty-four more amino acids. Then the pre-prodynorphin molecule comes to an end (as far as we know).

The June 13, 1983, issue of *Life Sciences* carried a report on new findings by Mitsuaki Suda and seven colleagues at the Kyoto University School of Medicine. Suda reported that this twenty-nine-amino-acid-long peptide, which he is calling leumorphin, showed strong opiate activity in the standard tests. Leumorphin has seventy times the opiate strength of Leu-enkephalin. Furthermore, leumorphin also interacts with the kappa opiate receptor. So do the other peptides which come from pre-prodynorphin— dynorphin and neo-endorphin.

Another interesting thing about leumorphin and its relation to dynorphin and pre-prodynorphin: dynorphin-24 is actually dynorphin-17 plus a Lys-Arg amino acid duo plus the initial Leu-enkephalin sequence of leumorphin. And dynorphin-32 is actually dynorphin-17 plus the Lys-Arg and the first thirteen amino acids in leumorphin. So apparently the body breaks these peptides at different places and for different reasons. The how is known—the peptides break at known cleavage points, amino acid duos such as lysine-arginine, arginine-arginine, and arginine-lysine. The why is still unclear. And in the case of dynorphin-32, there is still a "how" question. For the two amino acids in positions 14 and 15 in leumorphin are arginine and serine, which is not usually considered a cleavage signal.

In Chapter 6 we talked about the connections between endorphins and pain. One of the possible connections has to do with the so-called placebo effect. A neutral substance such as sugar water can produce in some people the same pain-killing effects as opiates like morphine. A 1978 experiment strongly suggested that this effect may be caused by endorphins. Placebo-sensitive people experience pain relief because their bodies make endorphins in response to their mental belief. The problem with the placebo-endorphin connection hypothesis has been that no experiments or clinical trials have confirmed the 1978 results.

In November 1983 researchers at the National Institute of Dental Medicine reported results that further complicate the issue. Richard Gracely and his co-workers gave dental patients hidden doses of either naloxone—the opiate antagonist—or a placebo. The placebo again produced pain relief in some of the subjects, and the naloxone again heightened the pain sensitivity of some subjects.

However, careful examination of the clinical trial's results showed that the effects of the placebo and the naloxone were independent of each other. In other words, the naloxone may well have been causing heightened pain sensitivity by blocking the action of the subjects' endorphins; but the placebo was *not* relieving pain by activating that same endorphin system. This in turn suggests that at least one non-opiate system is influencing pain perception. Scientists already know that Substance P plays an important role in nociception. There's also evidence that the neurotransmitters serotonin and norepinephrine may also be involved.

So the endorphin-placebo connection is probably not as straightforward as was once believed. In fact, it may not even exist.

Chapter 7 talked about connections between endorphins and drug abuse. An extremely interesting experiment performed in 1983 produced powerful evidence for such a connection. Jan Van Ree of the University of Utrecht in the Netherlands showed that certain endorphin fragments affected the self-administration of heroin in suitably trained experimental rats. In particular, the beta-endorphin fragment running from positions 2 through 9 (or Gly-Gly-Phe-Met-Thr-Ser-Glu-Lys) caused the rats to increase the dosage of heroin they were giving themselves. Another opioid peptide fragment known as DTgE (which we met in Chapter 8, "Endorphins and Mental Illness") did just the opposite: it caused the rats to decrease their heroin intake.

Ree's results, reported in the December 5, 1983, issue of *Life Sciences,* are most exciting. The DTgE effect could point the way to new methods of controlling heroin addiction. However, Ree's results with beta-endorphin could have more sinister consequences.

In Chapter 9, "Endorphins and Stress," we talked about the possible connections between endorphins and the immune system, which protects us from the onslaught of disease-causing organisms. In January 1984 researchers at UCLA reported a possible connection between endorphins, stress and the immune system.

Yehuda Shavit and four colleagues studied the effects of stress-causing foot shocks on the levels of endorphins and reduced resistance to disease in experimental rats. They discovered that certain patterns of foot shock seemed to cause the release of endorphins. That same pattern also caused a decrease in the effectiveness of the immune system cells called natural killer cells, or NK cells.

In another set of experiments, the researchers injected cancer-causing cells into rats given the foot shocks. Needless to say, some of the rats died of cancer. Some rats, though, who later got the endorphin-releasing foot-shock pattern and then the cancer cell injections, were first given injections of naltrexone, an opiate-blocking chemical. In these rats the rate of survival rose back to that in a non-stressed control group of rats.

The explanation for the findings? There are at least two. First, it is possible that endorphins released by foot-shock stress suppress immune function directly. There is already some other evidence that endorphins and morphine can affect immune function.

It is also possible that opioids like beta-endorphin affect NK cells indirectly. Endorphins may act to release or modulate the release of other hormones which do directly suppress the immune system's activity. One culprit might be ACTH. It is also known that morphine suppresses the release of interferon, which is known to increase the activity of NK cells. Perhaps endorphins also suppress the action of interferon. If that turns out to be the case, then we may here have the first glimmering of a linkage between two of the "hottest" biological substances of the last fifteen years, endorphins and interferon.

Chapter 10, "Other Endorphin Connections," includes a fascinating grab-bag of possible endorphin linkages. In 1983 several others came to light. They include possible connections between endorphins and SIDS, or Sudden Infant Death Syndrome, and Alzheimer's disease; and the effects of radiation on endorphin levels.

The endorphin-SIDS connection could be very important. In fact, it could be a causal connection. Aurelio Pasi and six colleagues at the University of Zurich did autopsies on two infants who died of SIDS. They found that both babies had apparently high concentrations of beta-endorphin and beta-lipotropin in their brainstems. Pasi used the word "apparently" on purpose—for no one yet really knows the *normal* levels of endorphins in the brains of infants. Pasi had to compare the levels he found with those in healthy human adults.

However, Pasi thinks that the levels he found were higher than normal. And he also believes that endorphins may be involved in causing SIDS. His theory is basically the same as that of Thomas Kuich and Donald Zimmerman of the Mayo Graduate School of Medicine. In 1981, Kuich and Zimmerman suggested that high levels of endorphins might be released in infants by the stress caused by innocuous (or not-so-innocuous) illnesses. Endorphins are known to suppress the breathing reflex and also the immune system. In the case of the cancer patients mentioned in Chapter 6 ("Endorphins and Pain"), endorphin injections even caused a loss of consciousness. Kuich and Zimmerman said it was possible that the high levels of endorphins might do the same thing in some babies. Their breathing reflex is super-depressed; the babies simply stop breathing.

Pasi agrees. He adds that pneumonia seems to be a common affliction in babies who die of SIDS. He thinks that high levels of endorphins interact with the life-threatening effects of pneumonia, and that this is the actual cause of SIDS. More work needs to be done to either confirm or kill the endorphin-SIDS theory. No doubt that work is going on now.

The endorphin-radiation connection is an interesting one, and is probably linked with the immune system. A group of researchers at the U.S. Air Force Academy found that laboratory mice exposed to radiation from cobalt-60 consumed less self-administered morphine than did a control group not exposed to the radiation. When the irradiated mice were given naloxone, which counteracts the effects of endorphins, they consumed more morphine. The researchers believe that the radiation caused an increase in endorphins in the mice, which in turn decreased their need for external opiates like morphine. The naloxone reversed the process, as would be expected of an opiate antagonist.

Another group of researchers at Massachusetts General Hospital (which included Daniel Carr, who did the endorphins-and-exercise study discussed in Chapter 9), looked at the levels of beta-endorphin and beta-lipotropin in the blood plasma of a man exposed to ultraviolet light. UV radiation, of course, is what causes suntans and sunburns. The researchers discovered that exposure to UV radiation caused a significant increase in endorphin and lipotropin in the man's blood.

Both results can be explained by the connection between endorphins and stress. Radiation can be stressful, particularly ionizing radiation from cobalt-60, which can cause damage to tissue. The body releases endorphins, among other chemicals, in response to stress. This seems also to be the case when the stressor is radiation.

In the case of the ultraviolet light, though, there is another explanation for the high levels of endorphins. When the skin is exposed to UV light it turns dark—it tans. Tanning is caused by an increase in skin pigmentation, which in turn is caused by an increase in the hormone called melanotropin. And where does melanotropin come from? Why, from the same precursor molecule for beta-endorphin and beta-lipotropin, that's where. Remember, the precursor's name is pro-opio*melano*cortin! The connection turns out to be simple: as the melanotropin is released to turn the skin darker, so is beta-endorphin. It's a side effect of tanning.

Several Japanese researchers in 1983 reported evidence of a decrease in beta-endorphin in the cerebrospinal fluid of people with Alzheimer's disease. This connection is not necessarily causal. Alzheimer's disease is characterized by serious loss of tissue in the frontal and occipital lobes of the brain. That is one of the major causes of the premature senility typical of Alzheimer victims. The decrease in beta-endorphin could be an effect of that loss of brain tissue. But the very fact that the decrease in beta-endorphin occurs is interesting. Does this decrease occur before any other symptoms of Alzheimer's crop up? That's not known. But if it does, then it may be possible to test people for incipient Alzheimer's by checking their cerebrospinal fluid levels of beta-endorphin.

The field of endorphin research continues—and will continue —to grow and flourish. Stay tuned. How? Well, almost none of the endorphin breakthroughs have been reported on television— it's hard to come up with exciting pictures. The weekly newsmagazines only occasionally carry a report or two on the field.

But you needn't travel far to keep up to date on the still breaking new waves of endorphin developments. Your local public and college libraries should have regular subscriptions to three magazines that will keep you in touch with the world of endorphins. They are *Nature*, *Science* and *Science News*. All three come out weekly. The first two contain actual research papers, but also have extensive and easy to understand news reports on all the scientific disciplines, including neuropharmacology. *Science News* is first, last and always "the weekly newsmagazine of science." There is nothing better around. If you can't find the first two, just read *Science News*. If you can't even find *Science News*, get a subscription. That way you can be sure of staying on top of the endorphin wave.

Olympia, Washington
23 January 1984

APPENDIX 1

A TIME LINE

A TIME LINE FOR THE
BRAIN AND ENDORPHINS

This time line, though not complete, lists some of the more important events in humanity's growing understanding of the brain. Information included here comes from numerous sources, including: Theodore H. Bullock, *Introduction to Nervous Systems* (W. H. Freeman, 1977); The Diagram Group, *The Brain: A User's Manual* (Putnam, 1982); *Information Please Almanac 1983* (Simon & Schuster, 1983) and primary reports in various scientific journals.

* * *

6th century B.C.—Pythagoras, the Greek philosopher who invented geometry's Pythagorean theorem, suggests the brain is the organ of the mind. This contradicts established belief, which holds the heart or the liver to be the seat of intelligence and views the brain as an organ for cooling the blood.

ca. 300 B.C.—Herophilus of Chalcedon, a Greek anatomist and surgeon, names the brain as the primary organ of the nervous system; he associates nerves with movement and feeling.

2nd century A.D.—Galen, a Greek physician, establishes incorrect theories of the brain that prevail for 1,500 years.

1543—Andreas Vesalius of Brussels, an anatomist, publishes the first modern anatomy of the brain.

1573—Constanzo Varoli, an Italian, illustrates the pons for the first time. Vesalius had missed it.

1660—Marcello Malpighi, an Italian anatomist, is one of the first people to use a microscope, specifically to study the brain.

1664—Thomas Willis, an English anatomist and physician, suggests the cerebellum in the brain governs involuntary movements and that thought takes place in the cerebrum.

1637—René Descartes, the famous French philosopher, states his belief that the soul is separate from the brain.

1691—Robert Boyle notes the existence of a motor cortex in the brain.

1730—Stephen Hales, an English physiologist, finds that reflex movements in frogs' legs depend on the spinal cord.

Late 1700s—Félix Vicq d'Azyr, a French royal physician, is one of the first people to note the wrinkled layers of the cerebrum in a preserved human brain.

1774—Domenico Cotugno, an Italian anatomist, declares that "animal spirit" does not fill the ventricles in the brain, but that cerebrospinal fluid does.

1791—Luigi Galvani, an Italian scientist, involuntarily stimulates the muscles of dissected frogs' legs with an electrical current.

1793—Philippe Pinel, a French physician, pioneers the humane treatment of people with mental illnesses. He was very much ahead of his time. We may still be behind his.

1809—Luigi Rolando, an Italian anatomist, suggests that the cerebrum controls deliberate acts, and the cerebellum controls involuntary functions. The fissure of Rolando is named for him.

1810—Franz Joseph Gall, a German physician, laid the basis for modern neurology with his dissections of brains and his remarkably modern suggestions about nerve organization. He was also one of the inventors of the pseudoscience of phrenology.

1811—Sir Charles Bell, a Scottish anatomist, theorizes that each nerve carries either a motor or a sensory stimulus, but not both at once.

Mid-1800s—Charles Brown-Sequard, a British physiologist and neurologist, makes numerous discoveries involving the spinal cord and the endocrine system which anticipate the discovery of neurotransmitters.

1837—Robert Remak, a German physician and physiologist, notes the true relation of nerve cells to nerve fibers.

1838—Johannes Purkinje, a Czech physiologist, describes a specific group of cells in the cerebellum, now known as Purkinje's cells.

1841—Hugo von Mohl, a German botanist, proposes that the inner contents of cells are not slime or moisture but a form of living matter he names protoplasm.

Late 1800s, early 1900s—Sir David Ferrier, a Scottish scientist, maps the region of the brain called the motor cortex and discovers the sensory strip.

1852—Hermann von Helmholtz, a German physicist, anatomist and physiologist, measures the speed of a nerve impulse in a frog.

1855—Bartolomeo Panizza, an Italian anatomist, shows that parts of the cerebral cortex are essential for vision.

1861—Paul Broca, a French surgeon and anthropologist, identifies a location in the left cerebral hemisphere which is associated with speech. It is now called Broca's area.

1865—In this year is published the first realistic drawing of a neuron.

1869—Friedrich Miescher, a German researcher, discovers deoxyribonucleic acid (DNA).

1873—Camillo Golgi, an Italian physician, devises a way to stain neurons so they show up under the microscope. It is now called the Golgi staining technique.

1874—Carl Wernicke, a German neurologist, discovers the area of the brain associated with understanding words. It is now called Wernicke's area.

1892—Sir Francis Galton, an English scientist, begins his pioneering scientific studies of the nature of intelligence.

1890s—Sigmund Freud is busy inventing psychoanalysis.

1898—John Newport Langley, an English physiologist, coins the term "autonomic nervous system."

1900—Max Planck, a German physicist, publishes his theory of the quantum.

1901—Santiago Ramón y Cajal, a Spanish histologist, demonstrates the true nature of the connections between nerves. The neurons don't touch; rather, the signal somehow jumps a "gap" now called the synapse.

—Jokichi Takamine, an American scientist, isolates the hormone epinephrine, eventually shown to be a neurotransmitter.

1904—Thomas Elliott, a British researcher, suggests that nerve impulses may be chemically transmitted.

1906—The first Nobel Prize in Medicine or Physiology to be awarded for work related to the brain goes to Santiago Ramón y Cajal and Camillo Golgi for their discoveries about the structure of the nervous system.

1909—Korbinian Brodmann publishes a map of the cerebral cortex giving numbers to different regions.

1914—John B. Watson, an American psychologist, proposes the theory of behaviorism.

Early 1900s—Keith Lucas, a British physiologist, establishes that stimulated neurons have an all-or-nothing response, much like that of the later-to-be-invented digital computer. This subsequently contributes to the vision of the brain as a computer, and computers as electronic brains.

1921—Otto Loewi, an American (German-born) pharmacologist, discovers that acetylcholine functions as a neurotransmitter. It is the first such chemical to be so identified.

Late 1920s—Wilder Penfield, a Canadian neurosurgeon, performs a series of brilliant experiments with microelectrodes to map areas of the human cerebral cortex.

1930—B. F. Skinner describes operant conditioning.

1932—Sir Charles S. Sherrington, an English physiologist, gets a Nobel Prize for his major work on inborn reflexes and his discoveries showing the central nervous system works at several different levels. He shares the prize with Edgar Douglas (Lord) Adrian, who did important research on the neuron.

1936—Otto Loewi gets the Nobel Prize for his 1921 acetylcholine discovery. He shares it with Sir Henry H. Dale, an English physiologist, who also has done major work on the nature of the chemical transmission of nerve impulses.

1944—A Nobel Prize goes to American physiologists Joseph Erlanger and Herbert Gasser for their work involving the amplification of nerve currents.

1947—A Nobel Prize is shared by Bernardo Alberto Housay of Argentina for his studies of the pituitary gland.

1949—Experiments involving probes of deep-brain functions with microelectrodes bring a Nobel Prize to physiologist Walter Hess of Switzerland.

—Giuseppe Moruzzi and Horace Magoun show that signals from the brain stem keep the whole brain awake.

1950—Philip Hench and Edward C. Kendall of the United States share the Nobel Prize in Medicine with Tadeus Reichstein of Switzerland for their discoveries concerning hormones of the adrenal gland.

—James Watson, Francis Crick and Maurice Wilkins discover the structure of DNA.

1955—Vincent du Vigneaud receives a Nobel Prize in Chemistry for his work on pituitary hormones.

1959—David Hubel and Torsten Wiesel publish research on how the brain interprets visual signals.

Late 1950s—Work by Vernon Mountcastle demonstrates that the neurons in the cortex are arranged in a million columns.

1961—Roger Sperry begins his work on the functions of "split brains" in humans.

—Roger Guillemin and Andrew Schally begin their attempts to discover hypothalamic hormones. Their collaboration eventually turns into competition.

1962—The discovery of the structure of DNA wins the Nobel Prize for Maurice Wilkins and Francis Crick of England and James Watson of the United States.

1963—Alan L. Hodgkin and Andrew Huxley of England and Sir John

Eccles of Australia get the Nobel Prize for their work on the mechanisms of nerve-impulse transmission.

1964—C. H. Li discovers a protein he later names beta-lipotropin.

1965—Li publishes the first (incorrect) structure of beta-lipotropin.

1967—A detailed account of the structure of the cerebellum is published by Janos Szentagothai and others.

1968—After seven years of work, Roger Guillemin (with Roger Burgus and Wylie Vale) announces the isolation of the first known hypothalamic hormone, TRF. Andrew Schally does also.

1969—Schally finds a second hypothalamic hormone, LRF. Guillemin moves from Baylor College of Medicine in Texas to the Salk Institute in California. He, too, finds LRF.

1970—A Nobel Prize goes to Julius Axelrod of the United States, Sir Bernard Katz of England and Ulf Svante von Euler of Sweden for research on neurotransmitters.

1971—A Nobel Prize goes to Earl W. Sutherland, Jr., of the United States for his work on how hormones function.

—Avram Goldstein suggests a new way to look for the binding sites for opiates which must exist somewhere on the neurons.

1972—Roger Guillemin and company isolate the third hypothalamic hormone, somatostatin.

1973—Candace Pert, Solomon Snyder, Eric Simon and Lars Terenius all discover the opiate receptor.

1975—The first known endogenous opioid peptide, enkephalin, is discovered nearly simultaneously by John Hughes of the University of Aberdeen, Scotland; Lars Terenius and Agneta Wahlstrom of the University of Uppsala, Sweden; and Solomon Snyder, Gavril Pasternak and Robert Goodman of the Johns Hopkins University School of Medicine of the United States. Primary credit usually goes to Hughes.

—Avram Goldstein and his associates announce the discovery of two other endogenous opioid substances which are not Hughes's enkephalin.

—John Hughes and Hans Kosterlitz later announce that enkephalin comes in two versions—namely, methionine-enkephalin (Met-enkephalin) and leucine-enkephalin (Leu-enkephalin)—and that the former is part of C. H. Li's beta-lipotropin.

1976—Roger Guillemin announces the discovery of alpha-endorphin.

—C. H. Li publishes the complete and correct amino acid sequence of beta-lipotropin.

—A. J. Kastin, Andrew Schally and others suggest that enkephalins can cross the "blood-brain barrier."

—C. H. Li and David Chung announce they have found a chemical in extracts of camel pituitary glands that is identical to amino acids 61–91 of beta-lipotropin, and which shows significant opiate-like activity. They have also made a synthetic version of it. They propose calling it beta-endorphin.

—A. F. Bradbury, D. G. Smyth and C. R. Snell report on work involving the so-called "C-fragment" (beta-endorphin) of beta-lipotropin.

—Avram Goldstein, C. H. Li and Brian Cox detail the way beta-endorphin acts like an opiate.

—Goldstein's first non-enkephalin opioid from 1975 is now known to be beta-endorphin. The second is still uncharacterized; he continues work on it.

—Seven Swiss researchers present evidence for the pain-killing activity of enkephalin in mice.

—Guillemin announces the discovery of gamma-endorphin.

—Guillemin, Larry Lazarus and Nicholas Ling suggest that beta-lipotropin is the precursor of the three endorphins (alpha-, beta- and gamma-) and the two enkephalins.

—Candace and Agu Pert, together with two other researchers, announce the creation of a synthetic enkephalin with extremely potent and long-lasting analgesic action in rats.

—P. J. Lowrey and two associates describe the presence of ACTH and beta-lipotropin within the same molecule.

—Two groups of researchers (Floyd Bloom, David Segal, Nicholas Ling and Roger Guillemin at the Salk Institute, and Yasuko Jaquet and Neville Marks at New York's Rockland Psychiatric Institute) demonstrate that injections of beta-endorphin cause cataleptic-type effects in mice.

—Psychiatrist Nathan Kline reports evidence from a small clinical test which suggests beta-endorphin can alleviate some symptoms of schizophrenia.

1977—Guillemin and Schally share a Nobel Prize for their pioneering work on hypothalamic hormones.

—Floyd Bloom pinpoints the location of endorphins in the pituitary gland.

—Li, Chung, Donald Yamashimo and Byron Doneen extract beta-endorphin from human pituitaries, and sequence it.

—British researchers Leslie Iversen and T. M. Jessell find that beta-endorphin and a synthetic version of Met-enkephalin strongly inhibit the release of Substance P in rat spinal nerves. Substance P is thought to be a pain neurotransmitter. Endorphins may help suppress pain.

—A research team led by Roger Nicoll of the University of California at San Francisco shows that endogenous opioid peptides seem to inhibit the actions of neurons in many brain regions. In the hippocampus, though, they excite the neurons. Results strongly suggest that endorphins and enkephalins are neurotransmitters, and that they may help regulate behavior.

—Richard Mains and Betty Eipper of the University of Colorado and Nicholas Ling of the Salk Institute report that a large protein called 31K-ACTH is almost certainly the precursor protein molecule of ACTH and the endorphins. They do not yet know its total amino acid sequence.

—Guillemin and seven collaborators report that beta-endorphin and ACTH are released at the same time by the pituitary.

—Three Finnish researchers find evidence for the presence of beta-endorphin in rat eye, pineal gland, kidneys, pancreas, gut and adrenal glands.

1978—Menachem Rubinstein, Stanley Stein and Sidney Udenfriend of the Roche Institute of Molecular Biology in New Jersey confirm that 31K-ACTH is the precursor to the endorphins and (they claim) Met-enkephalin. It is not a Leu-enkephalin precursor, though. They name it pro-opiocortin.

—A clinical study by Stanley Watson and others finds that naloxone causes a decrease in the hallucinations of schizophrenics. This points to an endorphin/schizophrenia connection.

—Udenfriend, Rubinstein, Stein and two others (Randolph Lewis and Louise Gerber) find two giant opioid-containing proteins in rat and guinea pig brains that are *not* pro-opiocortin.

—A Salk Institute team led by Bloom finds that beta-endorphin-containing circuits in rat brain are anatomically distinguishable from enkephalin-containing pathways.

—Floyd Bloom, Roger Guillemin, Jean Rossier and Yoshio Hosobuchi report that when pain in humans is relieved through electrical stimulation of part of their brains, the brain levels of beta-endorphin-like substances rise.

—Jon Levine, Newton Gordon and Howard Fields report that endorphins are implicated in the well-known placebo effect.

—Alan Faden and John Holaday report evidence that endorphins have an important role in traumatic shock.

1979—Japanese scientists Kenji Kangawa, Hisayuki Matsuo and Masao Igarashi announce the discovery of alpha-neo-endorphin. It contains a Leu-enkephalin sequence at its NH_2- terminal.

—Sidney Udenfriend, Randolph Lewis and several co-workers publish a number of reports in the course of the year on their discoveries of enkephalins, enkephalin-like peptides and larger opioid non-endorphin peptides in parts of animal adrenal glands.

—Four researchers at St. Elizabeth's Hospital in Washington, D.C., report that repeated electroconvulsive shocks (ECS), similar to those used to treat some mentally ill people, increase the levels of Met-en-kephalin in parts of the brain.

—Michel Chrétien suggests the endorphin/ACTH precursor be called pro-opiomelanocortin. Eventually the name is accepted and abbreviated to POMC.

—G. L. Belenky and John Holaday at Walter Reed Army Medical Center report evidence that endorphins are involved in the regulation of respiration and cardiovascular function during stress.

—Jean Rossier, Floyd Bloom and others find that genetically fat mice have abnormally high levels of Leu-enkephalin in parts of their brains.

—Des-Tyrosine-gamma-endorphin (DTgE) is found to be a possible "endogenous anti-schizophrenia" drug.

—Shigetada Nakashini and six colleagues determine the complete amino acid sequence of POMC via DNA cloning technology.

—British researcher Vicky Clement-Jones finds that successful electroacupuncture with heroin addicts is associated with a rise in Met-enkephalin levels in cerebrospinal fluid.

—Avram Goldstein determines the amino acid sequence of his second 1975 opioid peptide and names it dynorphin. Like alpha-neo-endorphin, it contains a Leu-enkephalin sequence at its NH_2- terminal.

1980—A clinical study by Philip Berger and others contradicts Kline's 1976 study with beta-endorphin and schizophrenics.

—The Roche Institute team discovers and determines the amino acid sequence for two possible enkephalin precursors, Peptides F and I.

—Goldstein studies "thrills" and finds a possible endorphin connection.

—Steven Gambert and three associates at the Medical College of Wisconsin produce data they think suggests that fasting is associated with decreases in hypothalamic beta-endorphin.

—Barbara Herman finds that dynorphin injected into the brains of rats makes them catatonic and causes profound analgesia.

—Tsutomu Oyama and four colleagues report dramatic pain-killing effects of beta-endorphin in people suffering from terminal cancer.

—E. T. Rolls announces that individual neurons deep in the brain seem to be associated with specific types of visual perception.

—S. I. Rapoport suggests that enkephalins may be able to cross the blood-brain barrier fairly easily.

—Lewis, Udenfriend and company announce in June the discovery of the enkephalin precursor. It contains seven copies of Met-enkephalin and one copy of Leu-enkephalin. However, they do not have an amino acid sequence determined for it.

—Three of the five researchers who did the study of endorphin anal-

gesia in terminal cancer patients report that beta-endorphin also induces rapid and prolonged pain relief in women giving birth.

—Dynorphin is found concentrated in parts of the pituitary gland, hypothalamus, medulla, pons, midbrain and spinal cord.

—Vicky Clement-Jones finds increased levels of beta-endorphin in the cerebrospinal fluid of people given acupuncture treatments for recurrent pain.

1981—Kangawa and Matsuo, with three others, publish the complete amino acid sequence for alpha-neo-endorphin and announce the discovery of beta-neo-endorphin, which is identical to alpha-neo-endorphin but lacks the final amino acid (a lysine).

—Two German researchers find evidence suggesting that the neurons in the frontal brain cortex of rats have multiple opiate receptors; i.e., more than one endorphin can plug into the same neuron simultaneously.

—Ray Moore and two associates at the University of Cambridge find a possible correlation between higher-than-normal levels of endorphins and anorexia nervosa.

—Three Canadian scientists publish a report implicating excessive production of endorphins in the development of abnormal menstrual conditions.

—Charles Denko of Fairview General Hospital in Cleveland suggests beta-endorphin is a culprit in rheumatoid arthritis.

—A detailed clinical study by Daniel Carr and others from Massachusetts General Hospital provides strong evidence of elevated levels of endorphins in runners and people doing exercise training.

—The Udenfriend team at Roche Institute detects and partially sequences the messenger RNA (or mRNA) for proenkephalin. They are close to breaking enkephalin's genetic code.

—Chavkin and Goldstein identify two specific amino acids inside dynorphin which make it possible for the peptide to plug into its particular receptor.

—Goldstein and his team announce that they have found the complete seventeen-amino-acid sequence for dynorphin.

—William Pardridge and Lawrence Mietus of the University of California at Los Angeles argue persuasively that the enkephalins do *not* get across the blood-brain barrier very well.

—Goldstein, Brian Cox and Lawrence Botticelli suggest that dynorphin in the spinal cord of mammals helps in the processing of sensory information.

—Jorge Mancillas of the University of California at San Diego, along with the Salk Institute people, find enkephalins and Substance P in the retina and eyestalk neurons of a lobster.

—A corticotropin-releasing factor (CRF) from sheep, forty-one amino acids long, is isolated, synthesized, and sequenced by a team including the Salk Institute's Wylie Vale. It releases beta-endorphin as well as ACTH.

—Nicholas Bodor of the University of Florida announces a way to sneak drugs across the blood-brain barrier.

—Eckard Weber, Kevin Roth and Jack Barchas show that alpha-neo-endorphin and dynorphin are contained in the same hypothalamic neurons.

—Roger Sperry shares a Nobel Prize for his "split-brain" work. Also sharing it are David Hubel and Torsten Wiesel for their work, initially published in 1959, on the brain and visual signals.

1982—The Roche Institute people refine their outline of the "biosynthetic pathway" that leads from proenkephalin to the enkephalins.

—Five researchers at Massachusetts General Hospital report that dosing rats with caffeine raises the levels of beta-endorphin in their blood.

—Ed Herbert and Michael Comb of the University of Oregon and Roberto Crea of Genentech, Inc., also report another partial reading of the mRNA of enkephalin.

—Between January and February 1982, three teams almost simultaneously report breaking the proenkephalin genetic code for both mRNA and cDNA (complementary DNA): the Roche Institute group with Udenfriend; the University of Oregon/Genentech group with Herbert and Comb; and a Japanese group led by Masaharu Noda. The Japanese group is given primacy of publication.

—Chavkin, Goldstein and Iain James suggest that dynorphin's receptor is the so-called "kappa" receptor.

—A team led by D. LeRoith and including Candace Pert finds beta-endorphin-like molecules inside a one-celled creature.

—Andrew Baird and others at the Salk Institute, including Guillemin and Ling, find evidence that the possible Met-enkephalin intermediate precursor BAM-12P may be present in the pituitary and the hypothalamus.

—Michael Boarder, Elizabeth Erdelyi and Jack Barchas find that large enkephalin-containing peptides circulate in the blood, along with enkephalins themselves and beta-endorphin. They, too, may be functioning as hormones and not merely as possible enkephalin precursors.

—Three researchers at the University of California at San Diego find that the brain chemical serotonin stimulates the release of beta-endorphin and ACTH. This is probably an important part of the body's response to stress.

—Robert Gerner and Burt Sharp of the University of California at Los Angeles report on a test for differences in the beta-endorphin levels in the cerebrospinal fluid of depressed, schizophrenic, anorexic or normal people: they find no significant differences.

—An opioid peptide similar to dynorphin is found in toad brains.

—Hitoshi Kakidani and nine colleagues, including Noda and Nakanishi, report the discovery and amino acid sequencing, via DNA cloning, of pre-prodynorphin. The precursor includes beta-neo-endorphin.

—Weber, Roth and Barchas find dynorphin and alpha-neo-endorphin co-located in still more places in the brain. They may be part of the same system. Some of these fiber systems seem to overlap systems already known to contain enkephalins.

—Several reports suggest a role for endorphins in the body's immune system.

—Burt Sharp and three associates at the University of California at Los Angeles show that dopamine helps regulate beta-endorphin levels in dogs.

—Goldstein and associates announce the discovery of dynorphin-23 and -32. Both contain two copies of Leu-enkephalin, and dynorphin-32 contains a new opioid peptide Goldstein names dynorphin-B. All are contained within pre-prodynorphin.

1983—A team of seven German researchers finds evidence for the presence of enkephalins in the heart. They surmise that enkephalins are involved in cardiac reflex mechanisms.

—The synthetic sheep CRF produced in 1981 by Wylie Vale and company is shown by him and his associates to stimulate secretion of beta-endorphin, ACTH and beta-lipotropin in human fetus pituitaries. This suggests, they say, that humans have a releasing factor in their hypothalami similar to that found in sheep.

—Alayne Yates, Kevin Leehey and Catherine Shisslak of the University of Arizona report on startling sociopsychological similarities between compulsive runners and anorexics. They suggest a possible role for endogenous opioids in both.

APPENDIX 2

---※---

LIST OF SOURCE MATERIAL

LIST OF SOURCE MATERIAL

This list of source material, arranged by chapters, includes both primary and secondary sources of information. Not all the books, research papers and news reports listed are specifically referred to in the text. However, they all constitute material that went into the eventual writing of this book.

Chapter 1   The Wonder of Our Stage
and
Chapter 2   A Peek Inside the Works

Adenohypophysis hormone. *McGraw-Hill encyclopedia of science and technology* 1:106–8. McGraw-Hill, 1982.

Bachelard, H. S. *Brain biochemistry.* Wiley, 1974.

Black, Ira B. Stages of neurotransmitter development in autonomic neurons. *Science* 215:1198–1204 (5 March 1982).

Bloom, Floyd, and Leslie L. Iversen. Localizing 3H-GABA in nerve terminal of rat cerebral cortex by electron microscopic autoradiography. *Nature* 229:628–30 (26 February 1971).

Brain barrier pierced. *Science Digest* 90:91 (December 1982).

Broadwell, R., et al. Morphologic effect of dimethyl sulfoxide on the blood-brain barrier. *Science* 217:164–67 (9 July 1982).

Bullock, Theodore H. *Introduction to nervous systems.* W. H. Freeman, 1977.

Burn, J. Harold. *The autonomic nervous system.* Blackwell Scientific Publications [London], 1976.

The Diagram Group. *The brain: a user's manual.* Putnam, 1982.

Eccles, Sir John C. *The physiology of the neuron.* Johns Hopkins Press, 1957.

———. *The understanding of the brain.* McGraw-Hill, 1973.

Fernstrom, John C., and Richard J. Wurtman. Nutrition and the brain. *Scientific American* 230:84–91 (February 1974).

Guyton, Arthur C. *Structure and function of the nervous system.* Saunders, 1976.

Iversen, Leslie L. The chemistry of the brain. *Scientific American* 241:134–49 (September 1979).

Lester, Henry A. The response to acetylcholine. *Scientific American* 236:106–20 (February 1977).

McEwan, Bruce S. Interactions between hormones and nerve tissue. *Scientific American* 235:48–59 (July 1976).

McIlwain, Henry, and H. S. Bachelard. *Biochemistry and the central nervous system.* Churchill Livingston [London], 1971.

Meltzer, Herbert L. *The chemistry of human behavior.* Nelson-Hall, 1979.

Nathanson, J. A., and P. Greengard. Second messengers in the brain. *Scientific American* 237:108–19 (August 1977).

The nature of brain function. Schering [n.d.].

The neurosciences: a study program. Rockefeller University Press, 1967.

Nicoll, Roger A. The interaction of porphyrin precursors with GABA receptors in the isolated frog spinal cord. *Life Sciences* 19:521–26 (15 August 1976).

———. Pentobarbitol: differential postsynaptic actions on sympathetic ganglion cells. *Science* 199:451–52 (27 January 1977).

———, and B. E. Alger. Synaptic excitation may activate a calcium-dependent potassium conductance in hippocampal pyramidal cells. *Science* 212:957–59 (22 May 1981).

———, and R. A. Jahr. Self-excitation of olfactory bulb neurons. *Nature* 296:441–44 (1 April 1982).

———, et al. Prolongation of hippocampal inhibitory postsynaptic potentials by barbiturates. *Nature* 258:625–27 (18 December 1975).

Pardridge, William M., and Lawrence J. Mietus. Enkephalin and the blood-brain barrier: studies of binding and degradation in isolated brain microvessels. *Endocrinology* 109:1138–43 (October 1981).

Patterson, Paul H., et al. The chemical differentiation of nerve cells. *Scientific American* 239:50–59 (July 1978).

Restak, Richard M. *The brain: the final frontier.* Doubleday, 1979.

Russell, Peter. *The brain book.* Hawthorne, 1979.

Shepherd, Gordon M. *The synaptic organization of the brain.* Oxford University Press, 1974.

Smith, Christopher U. M. *The brain: towards an understanding.* Putnam, 1970.

Smuggling drugs across the blood-brain barrier. *Science News* 121:7 (2 January 1982).

Taylor, Gordon Rattray. *Natural history of the mind.* Dutton, 1979.

Viannini, Vanio, and Giuliano Pogliani, eds. *The color atlas of human anatomy.* Beekman House, 1980.

Worden, Frederic G., et al., eds. *The neurosciences: paths of discovery.* MIT Press, 1975.

Chapter 3   The Discovery of the Endorphins

Arehart-Treichel, Joan. Winning and losing: the medical awards game. *Science News* 115:120, 126 (24 February 1979).

Birk, Yehudith, and Choh Hao Li. Isolation and properties of a new, biologically active peptide from sheep pituitary glands. *Journal of Biological Chemistry* 239:1048–52 (April 1964).

Bradbury, A. F., et al. C fragment of lipotropin has a high affinity for brain opiate receptors. *Nature* 260:793–95 (29 April 1976).

Chrétien, Michel, et al. A B-LPH precursor model: recent developments concerning morphine-like substances. *ACTH and related peptides: structure, regulation and action (Annals of the New York Academy of Sciences)* 27:84–107 (1977).

Comb, Michael, et al. Partial characterization of the mRNA that codes for enkephalins in bovine adrenal medulla and human pheochromocytoma. *Proceedings. National Academy of Sciences (U.S.A.)* 79:360–64 (January 1982).

———. Primary structure of the human Met- and Leu-enkephalin precursor and its mRNA. *Nature* 295:663–66 (25 February 1982).

Cox, Brian M., et al. Opioid activity of a peptide, B-lipotropin-(61–91), derived from B-lipotropin. *Proceedings. National Academy of Sciences (U.S.A.)* 73:1821–23 (June 1976).

———. A peptide-like substance from pituitary that acts like a morphine. 2. Purification and properties. *Life Sciences* 16:1777–82 (15 June 1975).

Dandekar, Satya, and Steven L. Sabol. Cell-free translation and partial characterization of proenkephalin messenger RNA from bovine striatum. *Biochemical and Biophysical Research Communications* 105:67–74 (15 March 1982).

DeRobertis, Eduardo. Molecular biology of synaptic receptors. *Science* 171:963–71 (12 March 1971).

Ehrenpreis, Seymour, et al. Approaches to the molecular nature of pharmacological receptors. *Pharmacological Reviews* 21:131–81 (June 1969).

Fischli, Walter, et al. Isolation and amino acid sequence of a 4000-dalton dynorphin from porcine pituitary. *Proceedings. National Academy of Sciences (U.S.A.)* 79:5435–37 (September 1982).

————. Two "big" dynorphins from porcine pituitary. *Life Sciences* 31:1769–72 (18–25 October 1982).

Ghazarossian, Vartan E., et al. A specific radioimmunoassay for the novel opioid peptide dynorphin. *Life Sciences* 27:75–86 (7 July 1980).

Goldstein, Avram, et al. Dynorphin-[1–13], an extraordinarily potent opioid peptide. *Proceedings. National Academy of Sciences (U.S.A.)* 76:6666–70 (December 1979).

————. Stereospecific and nonspecific interactions of the morphine congener levorphanol in subcellular fractions of mouse brain. *Proceedings. National Academy of Sciences (U.S.A.)* 68:1742–47 (August 1971).

Gubler, Ueli, et al. Detection and partial characterization of proenkephalin mRNA. *Proceedings. National Academy of Sciences (U.S.A.)* 78:5484–87 (September 1981).

————. Molecular cloning establishes proenkephalin as precursor of enkephalin-containing peptides. *Nature* 295:206–8 (21 January 1982).

Guillemin, Roger. Peptides in the brain: the new endocrinology of the neuron. *Science* 202:390–402 (27 October 1978).

————, et al. Characterization of the endorphins, novel hypothalamic and neurohypophysial peptides with opiate-like activity: evidence that they induce profound behavioral changes. *Psychoneuroendocrinology* 2:59–62 (1977).

————. The endorphins: novel peptides of brain and hypophysial origin, with opiate-like activity: biochemical and biologic properties. In: *ACTH and related peptides: structure, regulation and action (Annals of the New York Academy of Sciences)* 27:131–57 (1977).

Hughes, John. Isolation of an endogenous compound from the brain with pharmacological properties similar to morphine. *Brain Research* 88:295–308 (2 May 1975).

————. Opioid peptides and their relatives. *Nature* 278:394–95 (29 March 1979).

————, et al. Identification of two related pentapeptides from the brain with potent opiate agonist activity. *Nature* 258:577–79 (18 December 1975).

————. Purification and properties of enkephalin—the possible endogenous ligand for the morphine receptor. *Life Sciences* 16:1753–58 (15 June 1975).

Kakidani, Hitoshi, et al. Cloning and sequence analysis of cDNA for porcine B-neo-endorphin/dynorphin precursor. *Nature* 298:245–49 (15 July 1982).

Kangawa, Kenji, et al. A-neo-endorphin: a "big" Leu-enkephalin with potent opiate activity from porcine hypothalamus. *Biochemical and Biophysical Research Communications* 86:153–60 (15 January 1979).

————. The complete amino acid sequence of a-neo-endorphin. *Bio-*

chemical and Biophysical Research Communications 99:871–77 (15 April 1981).

Kilpatrick, Daniel L., et al. Rimorphin, a unique, naturally-occurring [Leu]enkephalin-containing peptide found in association with dynorphin and a-neo-endorphin. *Proceedings. National Academy of Sciences (U.S.A.)* 79:6480–83 (November 1982).

Kolata, Gina. Molecular biology of brain hormones. *Science* 215:1223–24 (5 March 1982).

Lazarus, Larry H., et al. Beta-lipotropin as a prohormone for the morphinomimetic peptides endorphins and enkephalins. *Proceedings. National Academy of Sciences (U.S.A.)* 73:2156–59 (June 1976).

Lewis, Randolph V., et al. An about 50,000-dalton protein in adrenal medulla: a common precursor of [Met]- and [Leu]enkephalin. *Science* 208:1459–61 (27 June 1980).

Li, Choh Hao. Lipotropin, a new active peptide from pituitary glands. *Nature* 201:924 (29 February 1964).

———, and David Chung. Isolation and structure of an untriakontapeptide with opiate activity from camel pituitary glands. *Proceedings. National Academy of Sciences (U.S.A.)* 73:1145–48 (April 1976).

———. Primary structure of human B-lipotropin. *Nature* 260:622–24 (15 April 1976).

Li, Choh Hao, et al. Isolation and amino acid sequence of B-LPH from sheep pituitary glands. *Nature* 208:1093–94 (11 December 1965).

———. Isolation, structure, synthesis and morphine-like activity of B-endorphin from human pituitary glands. In: *ACTH and related peptides: structure, regulation and action (Annals of the New York Academy of Sciences)* 27:158–66 (1977).

Ling, Nicholas, et al. Isolation, primary structure and synthesis of alpha-endorphin and gamma-endorphin, two peptides of hypothalamic-hypophysial origin with morphinomimetic activity. *Proceedings. National Academy of Sciences (U.S.A.)* 73:3942–46 (November 1976).

Mains, Richard E., et al. Common precursor to corticotropins and endorphins. *Proceedings. National Academy of Sciences (U.S.A.)* 74:3014–18 (July 1977).

Maisel, Merry, et al. Indignation over Pert affair [letter]. *Science News* 115:307 (12 May 1979).

Maran, Thomas H. Lasker Award and opiate receptors [letter]. *Science* 203:834 (2 March 1979).

Marx, Jean L. Lasker Award stirs controversy. *Science* 203:341 (26 January 1979).

Minimino, Naoto, et al. B-neo-endorphin, a new hypothalamic "big" Leu-enkephalin of porcine origin: its purification and the complete amino acid sequence. *Biochemical and Biophysical Research Communications* 99:864–70 (15 April 1981).

Nakanishi, Shigetada, et al. Nucleotide sequence of cloned cDNA for bovine corticotropin-B-lipotropin precursor. *Nature* 278:423–27 (29 March 1979).

Noda, Masaharu, et al. Cloning and sequence analysis of cDNA for bovine adrenal pre-proenkephalin. *Nature* 295:202–6 (21 January 1982).

The painkillers. *Time* 112:96 (4 December 1978).

Pasternak, Gavril W., et al. An endogenous morphine-like factor in mammalian brain. *Life Sciences* 16:1765–69 (15 June 1975).

Pert, Candace, and Solomon H. Snyder. Opiate receptor: demonstration in nervous tissue. *Science* 179:1011–14 (9 March 1973).

Pollin, William. More on medical awards [letter]. *Science News* 115:179 (24 March 1979).

Roberts, James L., et al. Corticotropin and B-endorphin: construction and analysis of recombinant DNA complementary to mRNA for the common precursor. *Proceedings. National Academy of Sciences (U.S.A.)* 76:2153–57 (May 1979).

Rubinstein, Menachem, et al. Characterization of pro-opiocortin, a precursor to opioid peptides and corticotropin. *Proceedings. National Academy of Sciences (U.S.A.)* 75:669–71 (February 1978).

Terenius, Lars. Stereospecific uptake of narcotic analgesics by a subcellular fraction of the guinea pig ileum. *Uppsala Journal of Medical Science* 78:150–52 (1973).

———, and Agneta Wahlstrom. Morphine-like ligand for opiate receptors in human CSF. *Life Sciences* 16:1759–64 (15 June 1975).

Teschemacher, H., et al. A peptide-like substance from pituitary that acts like morphine. 1. Isolation. *Life Sciences* 16:1771–76 (15 June 1975).

Chapter 4   Origins and Destinations

Boileau, Guy, et al. Biosynthesis of B-endorphin from pro-opiomelanocortin. In: *Hormonal Proteins and Peptides* 10:65–87 (1981).

Chavkin, Charles, and Avram Goldstein. Demonstration of a specific dynorphin receptor in guinea pig ileum myenteric plexus. *Nature* 291:591–93 (18 June 1981).

———. Specific receptor for the opioid peptide dynorphin: structure-activity relationships. *Proceedings. National Academy of Sciences (U.S.A.)* 78:6543–47 (October 1981).

Chavkin, Charles, et al. Dynorphin is a specific endogenous ligand of the k opioid receptor. *Science* 215:413–15 (22 January 1982).

Chrétien, Michel, et al. A B-LPH precursor model: recent developments concerning morphine-like substances. In: *ACTH and related peptides: structure, regulation and action (Annals of the New York Academy of Sciences)* 27:84–107 (1977).

Comb, Michael, et al. Partial characterization of the mRNA that codes for enkephalins in bovine adrenal medulla and human pheochromocytoma. *Proceedings. National Academy of Sciences (U.S.A.)* 79:360–64 (January 1982).

———. Primary structure of the human Met- and Leu-enkephalin precursor and its mRNA. *Nature* 295:663–66 (25 February 1982).

Corbett, Alistair, et al. Dynorphin (1–8) and dynorphin (1–9) are ligands for the k-subtype of opiate receptor. *Nature* 299:79–81 (2 September 1982).

Dandekar, Satya, and Steven L. Sabol. Cell-free translation and partial characterization of proenkephalin messenger RNA from bovine striatum. *Biochemical and Biophysical Research Communications* 105:67–74 (15 March 1982).

DeRobertis, Eduardo. Molecular biology of synaptic receptors. *Science* 171:963–71 (12 March 1971).

Ehrenpreis, Seymour, et al. Approaches to the molecular nature of pharmacological receptors. *Pharmacological Reviews* 21:131–81 (June 1969).

Fischli, Walter, et al. Isolation and amino acid sequence of a 4000-dalton dynorphin from porcine pituitary. *Proceedings. National Academy of Sciences (U.S.A.)* 79:5435–37 (September 1982).

———. Two "big" dynorphins from porcine pituitary. *Life Sciences* 31:1769–72 (18–25 October 1982).

Goldstein, Avram. Dynorphin and the dynorphin receptor: some implications of gene duplication of the opioid message. In: *Molecular genetic neuroscience,* ed. F. O. Schmitt, S. J. Bird and F. E. Bloom. Raven Press, 1982.

———. Minireview: opiate receptors. *Life Sciences* 14:615–23 (16 February 1974).

———. Stereospecific and nonspecific interactions of the morphine congener levorphanol in subcellular fractions of mouse brain. *Proceedings. National Academy of Sciences (U.S.A.)* 68:1742–47 (August 1971).

Gubler, Ueli, et al. Detection and partial characterization of proenkephalin mRNA. *Proceedings. National Academy of Sciences (U.S.A.)* 78:5484–87 (September 1981).

———. Molecular cloning establishes proenkephalin as precursor of enkephalin-containing peptides. *Nature* 295:206–8 (21 January 1982).

Hammonds, R. Glenn, et al. Characterization of B-endorphin binding protein (receptor) from rat brain membrane. *Proceedings. National Academy of Sciences (U.S.A.)* 79:6494–96 (November 1982).

Herbert, Edward, et al. Presence of a presequence (signal sequence) in the common precursor to ACTH and endorphin and the role of glycosylation in processing of the precursor and secretion of ACTH and endorphin. *Annals of the New York Academy of Sciences* 343:79–93 (1980).

Hook, Vivian Y. H., et al. A carboxypeptidase processing enzyme for enkephalin precursors. *Nature* 295:341–42 (28 January 1982).

Hoshima, H., et al. Rat pro-opiomelanocortin contains sulfate. *Science* 217:63–64 (2 July 1982).

Hudgin, R. L., et al. Enkephalinase: selective peptide inhibitors. *Life Sciences* 29:2593–2601 (21 December 1981).

Jones, Barry N., et al. Adrenal opioid proteins of 8600 and 12,600 daltons: intermediates in proenkephalin processing. *Proceedings. National Academy of Sciences (U.S.A.)* 79:2096–2100 (March 1982).

———. Enkephalin biosynthetic pathway: a 5300-dalton adrenal polypeptide that terminates at its COOH end with the sequence [Met]-enkephalin-Arg-Gly-Leu-COOH. *Proceedings. National Academy of Sciences (U.S.A.)* 79:1313–15 (February 1982).

———. Structure of two adrenal polypeptides containing multiple enkephalin sequences. *Archives of Biochemistry and Biophysics* 204:392–95 (1 October 1980).

Kakidani, Hitoshi, et al. Cloning and sequence analysis of cDNA for porcine B-neo-endorphin/dynorphin precursor. *Nature* 298:245–49 (15 July 1982).

Kilpatrick, Daniel L., et al. A highly potent 3200-dalton adrenal opioid peptide that contains both a [Met]- and a [Leu]enkephalin sequence. *Proceedings. National Academy of Sciences (U.S.A.)* 78:3265–68 (May 1981).

———. Identification of the octapeptide [Met]enkephalin-Arg[6]-Gly[7]-Leu[8] in extracts of bovine adrenal medulla. *Biochemical and Biophysical Research Communications* 103:698–705 (30 November 1981).

———. Release of enkephalins and enkephalin-containing polypeptides from perfused beef adrenal glands. *Proceedings. National Academy of Sciences (U.S.A.)* 77:7473–75 (December 1980).

Kimura, Sadao, et al. Probable precursors of [Leu]enkephalin and [Met]enkephalin in adrenal medulla: peptides of 3 and 5 kilodaltons. *Proceedings. National Academy of Sciences (U.S.A.)* 77:1681–85 (March 1980).

Lazarus, Larry H., et al. Beta-lipotropin as a prohormone for the morphinomimetic peptides endorphins and enkephalins. *Proceedings. National Academy of Sciences (U.S.A.)* 73:2156–59 (June 1976).

Lewis, Randolph V., et al. An about 50,000-dalton protein in adrenal medulla: a common precursor of [Met]- and [Leu]enkephalin. *Science* 208:1459–61 (27 June 1980).

———. Enkephalin biosynthetic pathway: proteins of 8000 and 14,000 daltons in bovine adrenal medulla. *Proceedings. National Academy of Sciences (U.S.A.)* 77:5018–20 (August 1980).

———. Opioid peptides and precursors in the adrenal medulla. In: *Neural peptides and neuronal communications,* ed. E. Costa and M. Trabucci. Raven Press, 1980.

———. Putative enkephalin precursors in bovine adrenal medulla. *Biochemical and Biophysical Research Communications* 89:822–29 (1979).

Li, Choh Hao. Lipotropin, a new active peptide from pituitary glands. *Nature* 201:924 (29 February 1964).

Li, Choh Hao, and David Chung. Primary structure of human B-lipotropin. *Nature* 260:622–24 (15 April 1976).

Liao, Chung Shin, et al. Evidence for a single opioid receptor type on the field stimulated rat vas deferens. *Life Sciences* 29:2617–22 (21 December 1981).

Mains, Richard E., and Betty A. Eipper. Biosynthetic studies on ACTH, beta-endorphin and alpha-melanotropin in the rat. *Annals of the New York Academy of Sciences* 343:94–110 (1980).

Mains, Richard E., et al. Common precursor to corticotropins and endorphins. *Proceedings. National Academy of Sciences (U.S.A.)* 74:3014–18 (July 1977).

Mizuno, K., et al. A new endogenous opioid peptide from bovine adrenal medulla: isolation and amino acid sequence of a dodecapeptide (BAM-12P). *Biochemical and Biophysical Research Communications* 95:1482–88 (29 August 1980).

———. A new family of endogenous "big" met-enkephalins from bovine adrenal medulla: purification and structure of docosa- (BAM-22P) and eicosapeptide (BAM-20P). *Biochemical and Biophysical Research Communications* 97:1283–90 (31 December 1980).

Nakanishi, Shigetada, et al. Nucleotide sequence of cloned cDNA for bovine corticotropin-B-lipotropin precursor. *Nature* 278:423–27 (29 March 1979).

Noda, Masaharu, et al. Cloning and sequence analysis of cDNA for bovine adrenal pre-proenkephalin. *Nature* 295:202–6 (21 January 1982).

Pert, Candace, and Solomon H. Snyder. Opiate receptor: demonstration in nervous tissue. *Science* 179:1011–14 (9 March 1973).

Pert, Candace, et al. Biochemical and autoradiographical evidence for type 1 and type 2 opiate receptors. In: *Neural peptides and neuronal communications,* ed. E. Costa and M. Trabucci. Raven Press, 1980.

Rackham, A., et al. Kyotorphin (tyrosine-arginine): further evidence for indirect opiate receptor activation. *Life Sciences* 30:1337–42 (19 April 1982).

Roberts, James L., et al. Corticotropin and B-endorphin: construction and analysis of recombinant DNA complementary to mRNA for the common precursor. *Proceedings. National Academy of Sciences (U.S.A.)* 76:2153–57 (May 1979).

Rossier, Jean, et al. Studies with [35-S]methionine indicate that the 22,000-dalton [Met]enkephalin-containing protein in chromaffin cells is a precursor. *Proceedings. National Academy of Sciences (U.S.A.)* 77:6889–91 (November 1980).

Rubinstein, Menachem, et al. Characterization of pro-opiocortin, a precursor to opioid peptides and corticotropin. *Proceedings. National Academy of Sciences (U.S.A.)* 75:669–71 (February 1978).

Simon, Eric J. Opiate receptors and endorphins: possible relevance to narcotic addiction. *Advances in Alcohol and Substance Abuse* 1:13–31 (Fall 1981).

————, et al. Recent studies on interaction between opioid peptides and their receptors. In: *Neural peptides and neuronal communication*, ed. E. Costa and M. Trabbuchi. Raven Press, 1980.

Smith, Andrew P., and Horace H. Loh. The opiate receptor. *Hormonal Proteins and Peptides* 10:89–170 (1981).

Snyder, Solomon H. Opiate receptors and internal opiates. *Scientific American* 236:44–57 (March 1977).

Stern, Alvin S., et al. Isolation of the opioid heptapeptide [Met]enkephalin[Arg[6], Phe[7]] from bovine adrenal medullary granules and striatum. *Proceedings. National Academy of Sciences (U.S.A.)* 76:6680–83 (December 1979).

————. Opioid hexapeptides and heptapeptides in adrenal medulla and brain: possible implications on the biosynthesis of enkephalin. *Archives of Biochemistry and Biophysics* 205:606–13 (December 1980).

————. Two adrenal polypeptides: proposed intermediates in the processing of proenkephalin. *Proceedings. National Academy of Sciences (U.S.A.)* 78:1962–66 (March 1981).

Terenius, Lars. Stereospecific uptake of narcotic analgesics by a subcellular fraction of the guinea pig ileum. *Uppsala Journal of Medical Science* 78:150–52 (1973).

Williams, J. T., and W. Zieglgansberger. Neurons in the frontal cortex of the rat carry multiple opiate receptors. *Brain Research* 226:304–8 (1981).

Wise, Steven P., and Miles Herkenham. Opiate receptor distribution in the cerebral cortex of the rhesus monkey. *Science* 218:387–89 (22 October 1982).

Zukin, R. Susan, and Steven R. Zukin. Minireview: multiple opiate receptors—emerging concepts. *Life Sciences* 29:2681–90 (28 December 1981).

Chapter 5   The Endogenous Opioid Peptides

Baird, Andrew, et al. Molecular forms of the putative enkephalin precursor BAM-12P in bovine adrenal, pituitary and hypothalamus. *Proceedings. National Academy of Sciences (U.S.A.)* 79:2023–25 (March 1982).

Bayon, A., et al. *In vivo* release of enkephalin from the globus pallidus. *Neuroscience Letters* 24(1):65–70 (1981).

Bloom, Floyd. Endorphins are located in the intermediate and anterior lobes of the pituitary gland, not in the neurohypophysis. *Life Sciences* 20:43–48 (1 January 1977).

————. Neuropeptides. *Scientific American* 245:148–68 (October 1981).

————, et al. Endorphins: developmental, cellular and behavioral aspects. In: *Neural peptides and neuronal communications*, ed. E. Costa and M. Trabucci. Raven Press, 1980.

————. Neurons containing B-endorphin in rat brain exist separately from those containing enkephalin: immunocytochemical studies. *Proceedings. National Academy of Sciences (U.S.A.)* 75:1591–95 (March 1978).

Boarder, Michael, et al. Opioid peptides in human plasma: evidence for multiple forms. *Journal of Clinical Endocrinology and Metabolism* 54:715–20 (April 1982).

Botticelli, Lawrence J., et al. Immunoreactive dynorphin in mammalian spinal and dorsal root ganglia. *Proceedings. National Academy of Sciences (U.S.A.)* 78:7783–86 (December 1981).

Chavkin, Charles, and Avram Goldstein. Demonstration of a specific dynorphin receptor in guinea pig ileum myenteric plexus. *Nature* 291:591–93 (18 June 1981).

Comb, Michael, et al. Primary structure of the human Met- and Leu-enkephalin precursor and its mRNA. *Nature* 295:663–66 (25 February 1982).

Cone, Ric I., and Avram Goldstein. A dynorphin-like opioid in the central nervous system of an amphibian. *Proceedings. National Academy of Sciences (U.S.A.)* 79:3345–49 (May 1982).

Cox, Brian M. Minireview: Endogenous opioid peptides—a guide to structures and terminology. *Life Sciences* 31:1645–58 (18–25 October 1982).

————, et al. Levels of immunoreactive dynorphin in brain and pituitary of Brattleboro rats. *Neuroscience Letters* 20:850–88 (1980).

Dockray, G. J., and R. G. Williams. Met-enkephalin-Arg(6)-Phe(7)-like immunoreactivity in the rat brain. *Journal of Physiology* 324:80P (March 1982).

Dupont, Andre, et al. B-endorphin and Met-enkephalins: their distribution, modulation by estrogens and haloperidol and role in neuroendocrine control. *Federation Proceedings* 39:2544–50 (June 1980).

Elde, R., et al. Immunohistochemical studies using antibodies to Leucine-enkephalin: initial observations on the nervous system of the rat. *Neuroscience* 1:349–51 (August 1976).

Fischli, Walter, et al. Isolation and amino acid sequence of a 4000-dalton dynorphin from porcine pituitary. *Proceedings. National Academy of Sciences (U.S.A.)* 79:5435–37 (September 1982).

————. Two "big" dynorphins from porcine pituitary. *Life Sciences* 31:1769–72 (18–25 October 1982).

Gibbs, D. M., et al. Synthetic corticotropin-releasing factor stimulates secretion of immunoreactive B-endorphin/B-lipotropin and ACTH by human fetal pituitaries *in vitro*. *Life Sciences* 32:547–50 (31 January 1983).

Goldstein, Avram, and Vartan E. Ghazarossian. Immunoreactive dynorphin in pituitary and brain. *Proceedings. National Academy of Sciences (U.S.A.)* 77:6207–10 (December 1980).

————, et al. Pituitary and brain opioid peptides (endorphins). In: *ACTH and related peptides: structure, regulation and action (Annals of the New York Academy of Sciences)* 27:108–14 (1977).

————. Porcine pituitary dynorphin: complete amino acid sequence of the biologically active heptadecapeptide. *Proceedings. National Academy of Sciences (U.S.A.)* 78:7219–23 (November 1981).

Guillemin, Roger, et al. B-endorphin and adrenocorticotropin are secreted concomitantly by the pituitary gland. *Science* 197:1367–69 (10 September 1977).

Horn, A. R. and J. R. Rodgers. Structural and conformational relationships between the enkephalins and the opiates. *Nature* 260:795–97 (29 April 1976).

Jones, Barry N., et al. Adrenal opioid proteins of 8600 and 12,600 daltons: intermediates in proenkephalin processing. *Proceedings. National Academy of Sciences (U.S.A.)* 79:2096–2100 (March 1982).

————. Enkephalin biosynthetic pathway: a 5300-dalton adrenal polypeptide that terminates at its COOH end with the sequence [Met]-enkephalin-Arg-Gly-Leu-COOH. *Proceedings. National Academy of Sciences (U.S.A.)* 79:1313–15 (February 1982).

————. Structure of two adrenal polypeptides containing multiple enkephalin sequences. *Archives of Biochemistry and Biophysics* 204:392–95 (1 October 1980).

Kakidani, Hitoshi, et al. Cloning and sequence analysis of cDNA for porcine B-neo-endorphin/dynorphin precursor. *Nature* 298:245–49 (15 July 1982).

Kilpatrick, Daniel L., et al. A highly potent 3200-dalton adrenal opioid peptide that contains both a [Met]- and a [Leu]enkephalin sequence. *Proceedings. National Academy of Sciences (U.S.A.)* 78:3265–68 (May 1981).

————. Release of enkephalins and enkephalin-containing polypeptides from perfused beef adrenal glands. *Proceedings. National Academy of Sciences (U.S.A.)* 77:7473–75 (December 1980).

Kimura, Sadao, et al. Probable precursors of [Leu]enkephalin and [Met]enkephalin in adrenal medulla: peptides of 3 and 5 kilodaltons. *Proceedings. National Academy of Sciences (U.S.A.)* 77:1681–85 (March 1980).

Land, R. E., et al. Evidence for the presence of enkephalins in the heart. *Life Sciences* 32:399–406 (24 January 1983).

Lazarus, Larry H., et al. Beta-lipotropin as a prohormone for the morphinomimetic peptides endorphins and enkephalins. *Proceedings. National Academy of Sciences (U.S.A.)* 73:2156–59 (June 1976).

LeRoith, D., et al. Corticotropin and B-endorphin-like materials are native to unicellular organisms. *Proceedings. National Academy of Sciences (U.S.A.)* 79:2086–90 (March 1982).

Lewis, Randolph V., et al. Enkephalin biosynthetic pathway: proteins of 8000 and 14,000 daltons in bovine adrenal medulla. *Proceedings. National Academy of Sciences (U.S.A.)* 77:5018–20 (August 1980).

————. High molecular weight opioid containing proteins in striatum. *Proceedings. National Academy of Sciences (U.S.A.)* 75:4021–23 (August 1978).

————. Opioid peptides and precursors in the adrenal medulla. In: *Neural peptides and neuronal communications,* ed. E. Costa and M. Trabucci. Raven Press, 1980.

————. Putative enkephalin precursors in bovine adrenal medulla. *Biochemical and Biophysical Research Communications* 89:822–29 (1979).

Li, Choh Hao, and David Chung. Primary structure of human B-lipotropin. *Nature* 260:622–24 (15 April 1976).

————, et al. Beta-endorphin—isolation, amino acid sequence and synthesis of the hormone from horse pituitaries. *International Journal of Peptide and Protein Research* 18(3):242–48 (1981).

————. Beta-endorphin: replacement of glutamic acid in position 8 by glutamine increases analgesic potency and opiate receptor-binding activity. *Biochemical and Biophysical Research Communications* 101(1):118–23 (1981).

Loh, Horace, H., and Choh Hao Li. Biologic activities of B-endorphin and its related peptides. In: *ACTH and related peptides: structure, regulation and action (Annals of the New York Academy of Sciences)* 27:116–30 (1977).

Mancillas, Jorge R., et al. Immunocytochemical localization of enkephalin and Substance P in retina and eyestalk neurons of lobster. *Nature* 293:576–78 (15 October 1981).

McGinty, Jacqueline F., et al. Dynorphin is contained within hippocampal mossy fibers: immunochemical alterations after kainic acid administration and colchine-induced neurotoxicity. *Proceedings. National Academy of Sciences (U.S.A.)* 80:589–93 (January 1983).

Mizuno, K., et al. A new endogenous opioid peptide from bovine adrenal medulla: isolation and amino acid sequence of a dodecapeptide (BAM-12P). *Biochemical and Biophysical Research Communications* 95:1482–88 (29 August 1980).

———. A new family of endogenous "big" Met-enkephalins from bovine adrenal medulla: purification and structure of docosa- (BAM-22P) and eicosapeptide (BAM-20P). *Biochemical and Biophysical Research Communications* 97:1283–90 (31 December 1980).

Nakanishi, Shigetada, et al. Nucleotide sequence of cloned cDNA for bovine corticotropin-B-lipotropin precursor. *Nature* 278:423–27 (29 March 1979).

Nicholas, P., et al. B-endorphin: opiate receptor binding activities of six naturally occurring B-endorphin homologs. *Proceedings. National Academy of Sciences (U.S.A.)* 79:2191–93 (April 1982).

Nicoll, Roger A., et al. Enkephalin blocks inhibitory pathways in the vertebrate CNS. *Nature* 287:22–65 (4 September 1980).

———. Neuronal actions of endorphins and enkephalins among brain regions: a comparative microiontophoretic study. *Proceedings. National Academy of Sciences (U.S.A.)* 74:2584–88 (June 1977).

Noda, Masaharu, et al. Cloning and sequence analysis of cDNA for bovine adrenal pre-proenkephalin. *Nature* 295:202–6 (21 January 1982).

Roberts, James L., et al. Corticotropin and B-endorphin: construction and analysis of recombinant DNA complementary to mRNA for the common precursor. *Proceedings. National Academy of Sciences (U.S.A.)* 76:2153–57 (May 1979).

Rossier, Jean, et al. Studies with [35-S]methionine indicate that the 22,000-dalton [Met]enkephalin-containing protein in chromaffin cells is a precursor. *Proceedings. National Academy of Sciences (U.S.A.)* 77:6889–91 (November 1980).

Rubinstein, Menachem, et al. Characterization of pro-opiocortin, a precursor to opioid peptides and corticotropin. *Proceedings. National Academy of Sciences (U.S.A.)* 75:669–71 (February 1978).

Siggins, George R., and W. Zieglgansberger. Morphine and opioid peptides reduce inhibitory synaptic potentials in hippocampal pyramidal cells *in vitro* without alteration of membrane potential. *Proceedings. National Academy of Sciences (U.S.A.)* 78:5235–39 (August 1981).

Stern, Alvin S., et al. Isolation of the opioid heptapeptide [Met]enkephalin[Arg[6], Phe[7]] from bovine adrenal medullary granules and striatum. *Proceedings. National Academy of Sciences (U.S.A.)* 76:6680–83 (December 1979).

———. Opioid hexapeptides and heptapeptides in adrenal medulla and brain: possible implications on the biosynthesis of enkephalin. *Archives of Biochemistry and Biophysics* 205:606–13 (December 1980).

———. Opioid polypeptides in guinea pig pancreas. *Proceedings. National Academy of Sciences (U.S.A.)* 79:6703–6 (November 1982).

———. Two adrenal polypeptides: proposed intermediates in the processing of proenkephalin. *Proceedings. National Academy of Sciences (U.S.A.)* 78:1962–66 (March 1981).

Sweetnam, Paul M., et al. Localization of immunoreactive dynorphin in neurons cultured from spinal cord and dorsal root ganglia. *Proceedings. National Academy of Sciences (U.S.A.)* 79:6742–46 (November 1982).

Viveros, O. Humberto, et al. Opiate-like materials in the adrenal medulla: evidence for storage and secretion with catecholamines. *Molecular Pharmacology* 16:1101–8 (1979).

Watson, Stanley J., et al. Dynorphin immunocytochemical localization in brain and peripheral nervous system: preliminary studies. *Proceedings. National Academy of Sciences (U.S.A.)* 78:1260–63 (February 1981).

———. Comparison of the distribution of dynorphin systems and enkephalin systems in brain. *Science* 218:1134–36 (10 December 1982).

———. Dynorphin and vasopressin: common localization in magnocellular neurons. *Science* 216:85–87 (2 April 1982).

———. Evidence for two separate opiate peptide neuronal systems. *Nature* 275:226–28 (21 September 1978).

Weber, Eckard, et al. Colocation of a-neo-endorphin and dynorphin immunoreactivity in hypothalamic neurons. *Biochemical and Biophysical Research Communications* 103:951–58 (15 December 1981).

———. Immunohistochemical distribution of a-neo-endorphin/dynorphin neuronal systems in rat brain: evidence for colocalization. *Proceedings. National Academy of Sciences (U.S.A.)* 79:3062–66 (May 1982).

———. Predominance of the amino-terminal octapeptide fragment of dynorphin in rat brain regions. *Nature* 299:77–79 (2 September 1982).

Williams, J. T. and W. Zieglgansberger. Neurons in the frontal cortex of the rat carry multiple opiate receptors. *Brain Research* 226:304–8 (1981).

Wise, Steven P., and Miles Herkenham. Opiate receptor distribution in the cerebral cortex of the rhesus monkey. *Science* 218:387–89 (22 October 1982).

Yang, H-Y.T., et al. Minireview: opioid peptides in adrenal gland. *Life Sciences* 27:1119–25 (September 1980).

Yoshimasa, Takaaki, et al. Methionine-enkephalin and Leucine-enkephalin in human sympathoadrenal system and phechromocytoma. *Journal of Clinical Investigation* 69:643–50 (March 1982).

Chapter 6   Endorphins and Pain

Abbata, D., et al. Beta-endorphin and electroacupuncture. *Lancet*, p. 1309 (13 December 1980).

Basbaum, Allan I. The modulation of pain: anatomical and physiological considerations. In: *Changing concepts of the nervous system*, ed. Adrian R. Morrison and Peter L. Strick. Academic Press, 1982.

————, and Howard L. Fields. Endogenous pain control mechanisms: review and hypothesis. *Annals of Neurology* 4:451–62 (November 1978).

————. Pain control: a new role for the medullary reticular formation. In: *The Reticular Formation Revisited*, ed. J. Allan Hobson and Mary A. B. Brazier. Raven Press, 1980.

Belluzi, James D., et al. Analgesia induced *in vivo* by central administration of enkephalin in rat. *Nature* 260:625–26 (15 April 1976).

Buscher, Heinz H., et al. Evidence for analgesic activity of enkephalin in the mouse. *Nature* 261:423–25 (3 June 1976).

Catlin, D. H., et al. Studies of beta-endorphin in patients with pain and drug addiction. *Hormonal Proteins and Peptides* 10:311–38 (1980).

Clement-Jones, Vicky, et al. Acupuncture in heroin addicts: changes in Met-enkephalin and beta-endorphin in blood and cerebrospinal fluid. *Lancet* II:380–83 (25 August 1979).

————. Increased beta-endorphin but not Met-enkephalin levels in human cerebrospinal fluid after acupuncture for recurrent pain. *Lancet* II:946–49 (1 November 1980).

Dias, P. L. R., et al. Effects of acupuncture in bronchial asthma: preliminary communication. *Journal of the Royal Society of Medicine* 75:245–48 (April 1982).

Endogenous opiates and their action. *Lancet* II:305–7 (7 August 1982).

Endorphins through the eye of a needle? *Lancet* I:480–82 (28 February 1981).

Evans, Frederick J. The placebo response in pain control. *Psychopharmacology Bulletin* 17:72–76 (April 1981).

Fields, Howard L., and Jon D. Levine. Biology of placebo analgesia. *American Journal of Medicine* 70:745–46 (April 1981).

Glazer, Ellen J., and Allan I. Basbaum. Immunohistochemical localization of Leucine-enkephalin in the spinal cord of the cat: enkephalin-containing marginal neurons and pain modulation. *Journal of Comparative Neurology* 196:377–89 (1981).

Glazer, Ellen J., et al. Serotonin neurons in nucleus raphe dorsalis and paragiganocellularis of the cat contain enkephalin. *Journal of Physiology* [Paris] 77:241–45 (1981).

Hameroff, Stuart R., et al. Doxepin effects on chronic pain, depression and plasma opioids. *Journal of Clinical Psychiatry* 43:22–26 (August 1982, sect. 2).

Han, J. S., and Lars Terenius. Neurochemical basis of acupuncture analgesia. In: *Annual review of pharmacology and toxicology* 22:193–220. Annual Reviews, Inc., 1982.

Hendler, Nelson. The anatomy and psychopharmacology of chronic pain. *Journal of Clinical Psychiatry* 43:15–20 (August 1982, sect. 2).

Herman, Barbara H., et al. Behavioral effects and *in vivo* degradation of intraventricularly administered dynorphin-[1-13] and D-Ala²-dynorphin-[1-11] in rats. *Life Sciences* 27:883–92 (1980).

Hill, R. G. Endogenous opioids and pain: a review. *Journal of the Royal Society of Medicine* 74:448–50 (June 1981).

Hosobuchi, Yoshio, et al. Elevation of beta-endorphin-like substance levels in the ventricular CSF by central gray stimulation (CGS) in humans. *Abstracts of the Society for Neuroscience*, no. A1293 (1980).

How does acupuncture work? *British Medical Journal* 283:746–48 (19 September 1981).

Huston, Barbara. Seattle obstetrician advocates return to nature's painkiller. Seattle *Post-Intelligencer*, p. C-7 (8 February 1981).

Janov, Arthur. *Prisoners of Pain*. Doubleday, 1980.

Jessel, T. M., and Leslie Iversen. Opiate analgesics inhibit Substance P release from rat trigeminal nucleus. *Nature* 268:549–51 (11 August 1976).

Levine, Jon D., et al. Mechanism of placebo analgesia. *Lancet* II:654–57 (23 September 1978).

Oyama, Tsutomo, et al. Beta-endorphin in obstetric analgesia. *American Journal of Obstetrics and Gynecology* 137:613–16 (1 July 1980).

———. Profound analgesic effects of beta-endorphin in man. *Lancet* I:122–24 (19 January 1980).

Pain, Theories of. *The new encyclopedia britannica* 13:865–67, 1982.

Pain. *McGraw-Hill encyclopedia of science and technology* 9:743–45. McGraw-Hill, 1982.

Pasternak, Gavril W. Opiate, enkephalin, and endorphin analgesia: relations to a single subpopulation of opiate receptors. *Neurology* 31:1311–15 (October 1981).

Pert, Candace B., et al. [D-Ala²]-Met-enkephalinamide: a potent long-lasting synthetic pentapeptide analgesic. *Science* 194:330–32 (15 December 1976).

Roques, B. P., et al. The enkephalinase inhibitor thiorphan shows antinociceptive activity in mice. *Nature* 288:286–88 (20 November 1980).

Toda, Kazuo. Response of raphe magnus neurons after acupuncture stimulation in rat. *Brain Research* 242:350–53 (24 June 1982).

Ulett, George A. Acupuncture treatments for pain relief. *Journal of the American Medical Association* 245:768–69 (20 February 1981).

Vaught, Jeffry L., et al. Mu and delta receptors: their role in analgesia and in the differential effects of opioid peptides on analgesia. *Life Sciences* 30:1443–55 (26 April 1982).

Wall, P. D., and C. J. Woolf. What we don't know about pain. *Nature* 287:185–86 (18 September 1980).

Chapter 7   Endorphins and Drug Abuse

Aghajanian, G. K. Central noradrenergic neurons: a locus for the functional interplay between alpha-2 adrenoceptors and opiate receptors. *Journal of Clinical Psychiatry* 43:20–24 (June 1982, sect. 2).

Bloom, Floyd, et al. Endorphins as mediators of ethanol actions: multidisciplinary tests. *Advances in endogenous and exogenous opioids: proceedings. July 26–30, 1981,* pp. 226ff.

Blum, Kenneth, et al. Reduced Leucine-enkephalin-like immunoreactive substance in hamster basal ganglia after long-term ethanol exposure. *Science* 216:1425–27 (25 June 1982).

Brady, Linda S., and Stephen G. Holtzman. Effects of intraventricular morphine and enkephalins on schedule-controlled behavior in nondependent, morphine-dependent and postdependent rats. *Journal of Pharmacology and Experimental Therapeutics* 219:344–51 (November 1981).

Catlin, D. H., et al. Clinical effects of B-endorphin infusions. In: *Neural peptides and neuronal communications,* ed. E. Costa and M. Trabucci. Raven Press, 1980.

————. Studies of beta-endorphin in patients with pain and drug addiction. *Hormonal proteins and peptides* 10:311–38. Academic Press, 1981.

Drug Addiction. *McGraw-Hill encyclopedia of science and technology* 4:395–96. McGraw-Hill, 1982.

Gaddis, Ronald R., and Walter R. Dixon. Modulation of peripheral adrenergic neurotransmission by methionine-enkephalin. *Journal of Pharmacology and Experimental Therapeutics* 221:282–88 (May 1982).

Gold, Mark, et al. Anti-endorphin effects of methadone. *Lancet* II:972–73 (1 November 1980).

Goldstein, Avram. *Principles of drug action.* Harper & Row, 1968; Wiley, 1973.

International Narcotics Research Club. *The opiate narcotics.* Pergamon Press, 1975.

Kantor, Robert E., et al. 5-Methoxy-*a*-Methyltryptamine (a,O-Dimethylserotonin), a hallucinogenic homolog of serotonin. *Biological Psychiatry* 15:349–52 (April 1980).

Koob, George F., et al. Effects of naloxone on the anticonflict properties of alcohol and chlordiazepoxide. *Substance and Alcohol Action/Misuse* 1:447–57 (1981).

Kuhar, Michael J. Receptors for clonidine in brain: insights into therapeutic actions. *Journal of Clinical Psychiatry* 43:17–19 (June 1982, sect. 2).

Milkman, Harvey, and Stanley Sunderwith. Addictive processes. *Journal of Psychoactive Drugs* 14:177–93 (July-September 1982).

Peterson, Robert C., and Richard C. Stillman, eds. *Phencyclidine (PCP) abuse: an appraisal.* NIDA Research Monograph 21. Department of Health, Education and Welfare, National Institute on Drug Abuse (August 1978).

Pickel, Virginia. Central noradrenergic neurons: identification, distribution and synaptic interactions with axons containing morphine-like peptides. *Journal of Clinical Psychiatry* 43:13–16 (June 1982, sect. 2).

Psychomimetic Drugs. *McGraw-Hill encyclopedia of science and technology* 11:77–79. McGraw-Hill, 1982.

Redmond, D. E., and Y. H. Huang. The primate locus coeruleus and effects of clonidine on opiate withdrawal. *Journal of Clinical Psychiatry* 43:25–29 (June 1982, sect. 2).

Simon, Eric J. Opiate receptors and endorphins: possible relevance to narcotic addiction. *Advances in Substance and Alcohol Abuse* 1:13–32 (Fall 1981).

Snyder, Solomon H. A multiplicity of opiate receptors and enkephalin neuronal systems. *Journal of Clinical Psychiatry* 43:9–12 (June 1982, sect. 2).

Stimmel, Barry, ed. *Opiate receptors, neurotransmitters and drug dependence: basic science—clinical correlates.* Hawthorne, 1981.

Tulunay, F. C., et al. Possible regulatory role of dynorphin on morphine- and beta-endorphin-induced analgesia. *Journal of Pharmacological and Experimental Therapeutics* 219(2):296–98 (1981).

Waterfield, Angela A., et al. Cross tolerance between morphine and methionine-enkephalin. *Nature* 260:624–25 (15 April 1976).

Wei, Eddie. Enkephalin analogs and physical dependence. *Journal of Pharmacology and Experimental Therapeutics* 216:12–18 (June 1981).

———, and Horace Loh. Physical dependence on opiate-like peptides. *Science* 193: 1262–63 (24 September 1976).

Yoshimura, Kohji, et al. Kappa opioid properties of dynorphin and its peptide fragments on the guinea pig ileum. *Journal of Pharmacology and Experimental Therapeutics* 222:71–79 (July 1982).

Chapter 8   Endorphins and Mental Illness

Barchas, Jack D. Opioid agonists and antagonists in schizophrenia. In: *Neural peptides and neuronal communications,* ed. E. Costa and M. Trabucci. Raven Press, 1980.

Belenky, G. L., and J. W. Holaday. The opiate antagonist naloxone modifies the effects of electroconvulsive shock (ECS) on respiration, blood pressure and heart rates. *Brain Research* 177:414–17 (1979).

Berger, Philip A. Behavioral pharmacology of the endorphins. In: *Annual review of medicine* 3:397–415. Annual Reviews, Inc., 1982.

———. Biochemistry and the schizophrenias. *Journal of Nervous and Mental Disease* 169:90–99 (February 1982).

———, et al. The effects of naloxone in chronic schizophrenia. *American Journal of Psychiatry* 138:913–18 (July 1981).

———, and Jack D. Barchas. Studies of beta-endorphin in patients with mental illness. *Hormonal Proteins and Peptides* 10:293–310 (1981).

Bloom, Floyd, et al. Endorphins: profound behavioral effects in rats suggest new etiological factors in mental illness. *Science* 194:630–33 (7 November 1976).

Catlin, D. H., et al. Clinical effects of B-endorphin infusions. In: *Neural peptides and neuronal communications,* ed. E. Costa and M. Trabucci. Raven Press, 1980.

Davis, Glenn, and W. E. Bunney, Jr. Psychopathology and endorphins. In: *Neural peptides and neuronal communications,* ed. E. Costa and M. Trabucci. Raven Press, 1980.

Gerner, Robert H., and T. Yamada. Altered neuropeptide concentrations in cerebrospinal fluid and psychiatric patients. *Brain Research* 238:298–302 (22 April 1982).

Gerner, Robert H., and B. Sharp. CSF B-endorphin-immunoreactivity in normal, schizophrenic, depressed, manic and anorexic subjects. *Brain Research* 237:244–47 (8 April 1982).

Herman, Barbara H., and Avram Goldstein. Cataleptic effects of dynorphin-[1-13] in rats made tolerant to a *mu* opiate receptor agonist. *Neuropeptides* 2:13–22 (1982).

Hong, J. S., et al. Repeated electroconvulsive shocks and the brain content of endorphins. *Brain Research* 177:273–78 (1979).

Jacquet, Yasuko F., and N. Marks. The C-fragment of B-lipotropin: an endogenous neuroleptic or antipsychotogen? *Science* 194:632–35 (5 November 1976).

Meltzer, Herbert Y., et al. Effect of Des-Tyr-γ-endorphin in schizophrenia. *Psychopharmacology Bulletin* 18:44–47 (January 1982).

Pedigo, N. W., et al. Possible role of opiate receptors and Des-Tyrosine-γ-endorphin in schizophrenia. In: *Neural peptides and neuronal communications,* ed. E. Costa and M. Trabucci. Raven Press, 1980.

Schizophrenia. *McGraw-Hill encyclopedia of science and technology* 12:105. McGraw-Hill, 1982.

Snyder, Solomon H. *Biological aspects of mental disorder.* Oxford University Press, 1980.

Verebey, Karl, ed. *Opioids in mental illness (Annals of the New York Academy of Sciences).* Vol. 398. New York Academy of Sciences, 1982.

Chapter 9   Endorphins and Stress

Carr, Daniel B., et al. Physical conditioning facilitates the exercise-induced secretion of B-endorphin and B-lipotropin in women. *New England Journal of Medicine* 305:560–63 (3 September 1981).

Exercise and the endogenous opioids [four letters to the editor]. *New England Journal of Medicine* 305:1590–92 (24 December 1981).

Holaday, John W., and Alan Faden. Naloxone treatment in shock. *Lancet,* p. 201 (25 July 1981).

Holaday, John W., et al. Hypophysectomy alters cardiorespiratory variables: central effects of pituitary endorphins in shock. *American Journal of Physiology* 241:H479–85 (October 1981).

————. Thyrotropin-releasing hormone improves blood pressure and survival in endotoxic shock. *European Journal of Pharmacology* 74:101–5 (September 1981).

Pert, Agu. The body's own tranquilizers. *Psychology Today,* 15:100 (September 1981).

Pardridge, William M., and Lawrence J. Mietus. Enkephalin and the blood-brain barrier—studies of binding and degradation in isolated brain microvessels. *Endocrinology* 109:1138–43 (October 1981).

Proulx Ferland, Louise, et al. Corticotropin-releasing factor stimulates secretion of melanocyte-stimulating hormone from rat pituitary. *Science* 217:62–63 (2 July 1982).

Rossier, Jean, et al. On the mechanisms of the simultaneous release of immunoreactive B-endorphin, ACTH, and prolactin by stress. In: *Neural peptides and neuronal communications,* ed. E. Costa and M. Trabucci. Raven Press, 1980.

Selye, Hans. *The stress of life.* McGraw-Hill, 1978.

Smuggling drugs across brain border. *Science News* 121:7 (2 January 1982).

Tortella, Frank C., et al. Opiate-like electroencephalographic and behavioral effects of electroconvulsive shock in rats. *European Journal of Pharmacology* 76:121–28 (December 1981).

Treichel, Joan A. Now brain proteins fight disease. *Science News* 122:55 (24 July 1982).

Yanagida, Hisashi, and Guenter Corssen. Respiratory distress and B-endorphin-like immunoreactivity in humans. *Anesthesiology* 55:515–19 (November 1981).

Yates, Alayne, et al. Running—an analogue of anorexia? *New England Journal of Medicine* 308:251–55 (2 February 1983).

Chapter 10   Other Endorphin Connections

Arnold, Michael A., et al. Caffeine stimulates B-endorphin release in blood but not in cerebrospinal fluid. *Life Sciences* 31:1017–24 (6 September 1982).

Bajorak, J. G., et al. Effects of B-endorphin on experimentally induced seizures in mice. *Proceedings. Western Pharmacological Society* 24:315–17 (1981).

Beta-endorphin as arthritis culprit. *Science News* 119:358–59 (6 June 1981).

Blankstein, J., et al. Endorphins and the regulation of the human menstrual cycle. *Clinical Endocrinology* 14:287–94 (March 1981).

Broadwell, R., et al. Morphologic effect of dimethyl sulfoxide on the blood-brain barrier. *Science* 217:164–67 (9 July 1982).

Einhorn, Daniel, et al. Hypotensive effect of fasting: possible involvement of the sympathetic nervous system and endogenous opiates. *Science* 217:727–29 (20 August 1982).

Ettenbenberg, A., et al. Endogenous opiates and fasting. *Science* 213:1282 (1981).

Goldstein, Avram. Thrills in response to music and other stimuli. *Physiological Psychology* 8(1):126–29 (1980).

Hernandez, L., and D. A. Powell. Effects of naloxone on Pavlovian conditioning of eyeblink and head rate responses in rabbits. *Life Sciences* 27:863–65 (8 September 1980).

Julliard, Jacques H., et al. High-molecular-weight immunoreactive B-endorphin in extracts of human placenta is a fragment of immunoglobin G. *Science* 208:183–85 (11 April 1980).

Koob, George F., and Floyd E. Bloom. Behavioral effects of neuropeptides: endorphins and vasopressin. In: *Annual review of physiology, 1982.* Annual Reviews, Inc., 1982.

Kosterlitz, Hans W. Possible functions of the enkephalins. In: *Neural peptides and neuronal communications,* ed. E. Costa and M. Trabucci. Raven Press, 1980.

Moore, R., et al. Naloxone in the treatment of anorexia nervosa: effect on weight gain and lipolysis. *Journal of the Royal Society of Medicine* 74:129–31 (February 1981).

Prezwlocki, R., et al. The opioid peptide dynorphin, circadian rhythms and starvation. *Science* 219:71–73 (7 January 1983).

Rossier, Jean, et al. Opioid peptides and a-melanocyte-stimulating hormone in genetically obese *(ob/ob)* mice during development. *Proceedings. National Academy of Sciences (U.S.A.)* 76:2077–80 (April 1979).

Squire, Larry R., and Hasker P. Davis. The pharmacology of memory: a neurobiological perspective. In: *Annual review of pharmacy and toxicology, 1981.* Annual Reviews, Inc., 1981.

Walker, J. Michael, et al. Nonopiate effects of dynorphin and Des-1yr-dynorphin. *Science* 218:1136–38 (10 December 1982).

Wong, T. M., et al. Beta-endorphin—vasodilating effect on the microcirculatory system of hamster cheek pouch. *International Journal of Peptide and Protein Research* 18(4):420–22 (1981).

Yates, Alayne, et al. Running—an analogue of anorexia? *New England Journal of Medicine* 308:251–55 (2 February 1983).

Chapter 11   The Endorphin Business

Abelson, Philip, ed. [Biotechnology issue]. *Science* (11 February 1983).

Anderson, Wayne. Biotechnology will be a major factor in crop farming. *Feedstuffs*, p. 8 (20 December 1982).

Biotechnology equipment sales rising. *Chemical and Engineering News* 60.22 (6 September 1982).

Biotechnology—seeking the right corporate combinations. *Chemical Week* 129:36–40 (30 September 1981).

Chisholm, Rex. On the trail of the magic bullet. *High Technology* 3:57–63 (January 1983).

Geller, Irving. Business outlook: biotechnology products. *High Technology* 3:60 (February 1983).

Gestation blues. *The Economist* 284:76–77 (31 July 1982).

Hochhauser, Steven J. Bringing biotechnology to market. *High Technology* 3:55–60 (February 1983).

Marx, Jean L. Still more about gene transfer. *Science* 218:459–60 (29 October 1982).

A shaky start for genetic engineering's first drug? *The Economist* 284:103–4 (25 September 1982).

Shine, John, et al. Expression of clone beta-endorphin gene sequences by *Escherichia coli. Nature* 285:456–61 (12 June 1980).

Stinson, Steve. Researchers synthesize custom-made gene. *Chemical and Engineering News* 60:19 (2 August 1982).

Study pessimistic on outlook for genetic engineering. *Journal of Commerce*, pp. 3A, 22B (8 December 1982).

U.S. biotechnology transfer policy being studied. *Chemical and Engineering News* 61:25–28 (17 January 1983).

Chapter 12   Beyond Endorphins

Blakemore, Colin. *Mechanics of the mind.* Cambridge University Press, 1977.

Calder, Nigel. *The mind of man.* Viking Press, 1970.

Eccles, Sir John C. Beyond the brain. *OMNI* 5:57–62 (October 1982).

———. *Facing reality.* Springer-Verlag, 1970.

Harth, Erich. *Windows on the mind: reflections on the physical basis of consciousness.* William Morrow, 1982.

Johnston, William. *Silent music: the science of meditation.* Harper & Row, 1974.

Kolata, Gina. Brain receptors for appetite discovered. *Science* 218:460–61 (29 October 1982).

Penfield, Wilder. *The mystery of the mind.* Princeton University Press, 1975.

Popper, Sir Karl, and Sir John C. Eccles. *The self and its brain.* Springer International, 1977.

Rieber, Robert, ed. *Body and mind: past, present, and future.* Academic Press, 1980.

Wolf, Fred Alan. *Taking the quantum leap: the new physics for nonscientists.* Harper & Row, 1981.

Afterword: Recent Developments

Bloom, Floyd E. The endorphins: a growing family of pharmacologically pertinent peptides. In: *Annual review of pharmacology and toxicology* 32:151–70. Annual Reviews, Inc., 1983.

Emrich, H. M., et al. Heroin addiction: beta-endorphin immunoreactivity in plasma increases during withdrawal. *Pharmacopsychiatra* 16:93–96 (May 1983).

Herbert, Wray. Placebo: killing pain without opiates. *Science News* 124:359 (3 December 1983).

Kaiya, H., et al. Decreased level of beta-endorphin-like immunoreactivity in cerebrospinal fluid of patients with senile dementia of Alzheimer type. *Life Sciences* 33:1039–43 (12 September 1983).

Levins, Paul C., et al. Plasma B-endorphin and B-lipotropin response to ultraviolet radiation. *Lancet* II:166 (16 July 1983).

Lightman, Stafford L., et al. Evidence for opiate receptors on pitui-cytes. *Nature* 305:235–37 (15 September 1983).

Matsuo, Hisayuki, et al. Novel C-terminally amidated peptide in human phaeochromocytoma tumor. *Nature* 305:721–23 (20 October 1983).

Meisenberg, Gerhard, and William H. Simmons. Minireview: peptides and the blood-brain barrier. *Life Sciences* 32:2611–23 (6 June 1983).

Mickley, G. Andrew, et al. Changes in morphine self-administration after exposure to ionizing radiation: evidence for the involvement of endorphins. *Life Sciences* 33:711–18 (22 August 1983).

Miller, Julie Ann. Opiate role in stress effect on immunity. *Science News* 122:332 (20 November 1982).

Pasi, A., et al. Regional levels of beta-lipotropin and beta-endorphin in the brain and hypophysis of victims of sudden infant death syndrome. *Archives of Pathology and Laboratory Medicine* 107:336–37 (June 1983).

Porreca, Frank, and Thomas F. Burks, eds. *Proceedings of the 1983 International Narcotic Research Conference.* Life Sciences 33, Supplement 1. 781 pp. (1983).

Shavit, Yehuda, et al. Opioid peptides mediate the suppressive effect of stress on natural killer cell cytotoxicity. *Science* 223:188–90 (13 January 1984).

Steinberg, Sara. Endorphins: new types and sweet links. *Science News* 124:136 (27 August 1983).

Suda, Mitsuaki, et al. A novel opioid peptide, leumorphin, acts as an agonist at the k opiate receptor. *Life Sciences* 32:2769–70 (13 June 1983).

van Ree, Jan. The influence of neuropeptides related to pro-opiomela-nocortin on acquisition of heroin self-administration in rats. *Life Sciences* 33:2283–90 (5 December 1983).